!!!

Frank Butterfield has trained groups and individuals in 18 countries and traveled around the world speaking on topics from personal motivation to training and instructing. He has served as chairman of the Professional Development Committee for ACE, taught as adjunct faculty at Clark County Community College, and been quoted by *Men's Fitness, Club Industry Today,* and *ACE Certified News.* Butterfield is a coach, fitness instructor, personal trainer, and member of the Advisory Board at the Las Vegas Athletic Clubs.

Mark Cibrario, C.S.C.S., is owner of The Trainers Club, a personal training studio in Northbrook, Ill., and serves as a consultant to SPRI Products and Harbinger. He is an NSCA- and ACE-certified Personal Trainer, a certified strength conditioning specialist through the NSCA, and a level 2 CHEK practitioner. Cibrario has co-produced 10 videos on strength training, authored two books for SPRI Products, and written on topics including program design for strength training, injury prevention, and post-injury fitness.

Sabrena Newton, M.S., has been actively involved in the fitness industry since 1987, focusing on teaching group exercise, owning and operating her own personal training business, and managing fitness departments in commercial fitness facilities. Newton is a former full-time faculty member in the kinesiology and physical education department at California State University at Long Beach. She has a bachelor's degree in exercise science as well as a master's degree in physical education from the University of Kansas, and has numerous certifications in exercise instruction. Newton, an ACE-certified Personal Trainer and Group Fitness Instructor, also educates other fitness professionals about current industry topics through speaking engagements at local establishments and national conferences.

CONTENTS

The American Council on Exercise (ACE) is pleased to introduce *Group Strength Training,* Second Edition, a guide for fitness professionals. This new edition features additional modifications for many exercises and an increased focus on client safety. For group fitness instructors, guidelines have been added to help you welcome new participants into the class setting. It is ACE's goal to establish guidelines and criteria so that this exercise modality can be practiced both safely and effectively. The intent of this book is to educate and give guidance to fitness professionals that wish to teach group strength training.

As with all areas of fitness, education is a continual process. ACE recognizes this is a broad subject requiring serious study and we encourage you to use the References and Suggested Reading to further your knowledge.

INTRODUCTION

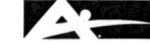

Introduction

C H A P T E R O N E

to Group Strength Training

G roup **strength training** instructors are challenged with teaching safe and effective exercise classes that will keep participants active and healthy.

Strictly adhere to the following guidelines to ensure a safe, effective, and fun strength-training class.

1. Perform all exercises slowly and with control. When exercises are performed too quickly or without maintaining proper form, there is a greater opportunity for injury. Also, music selection should reflect the need to keep the speed of the movement slow and controlled.

2. Know your participants' needs and health histories. It is difficult to give the participants what they want unless you clearly understand their needs and limits. Ideally,

participants should have completed a health-history form and listed their goals prior to participating.

3. Choose exercises that can be modified for participants at all levels of fitness. In a group setting, modifications to exercises must be offered to allow for individual differences. Whenever possible, teach to the high-average level of the class and provide modifications for intensity and skill level.

4. To realize improvements in **muscular strength,** repetitions should be kept relatively low (8–12) whenever possible. By keeping the weight high and the repetitions low, participants can continue to benefit from the progressive nature of strength training. Remember that new participants will benefit from performing higher repetitions with less resistance for the first few weeks.

5. Stretch targeted muscle groups before and after the workout. Proper stretching helps maintain muscles that are pliable and healthy, with the greatest benefits derived from stretching after the workout.

6. Give specific feedback to help improve performance. Participants need to know what they are doing correctly and how to improve their performance. In some cases, participants may copy form incorrectly modeled by another participant.

7. Create clear instructions to safely and effectively teach participants correct form. Use words that have meaning to participants and use both verbal and visual communication techniques.

8. Transition from one exercise to another using small changes. Avoid sequencing exercises in a way that wastes time due to equipment changes. Likewise, avoid moving your participants back and forth from a standing to lying position.

9. Acknowledge all participants and help them feel like part of the group. Learn names and introduce new participants to regular class attendees. Make eye contact with each participant a minimum of three times per class. Treat first timers with extra special care, make them feel welcome, and encourage them to come back for a second class.

10. Make the class fun.

History

The development of group strength training has undergone four distinct phases. Group strength training initially began as group **calisthenics.** Exercises were simple and equipment was scarce. Classes were offered as part of sports team training or physical education. A typical class included sit-ups, push-ups, and squats. Exercises were selected with little attention to safety, and modifications were rarely offered.

During the next phase, group strength training developed in health clubs as group exercise classes. The emphasis of the classes was on high repetitions and "feeling the burn." Participants

were attracted to the misconception that high-repetition exercises burned fat, spot reduced, or somehow slimmed the body. Exercise selection was diverse and, although attention was paid to form, safety and effectiveness were lacking.

During the third phase of group strength training, more attention was paid to safety and effectiveness. Traditional exercises (e.g., full sit-ups) were excluded and limits were placed on controversial movements such as forward **flexion** and deep knee flexion. A greater variety of exercise equipment became available, creating program diversity. The number of repetitions was reduced as the emphasis shifted from endurance training to strength training.

In the most recent phase, classes emphasize functional strength training along with a greater diversity of exercises, formats, and equipment. Also, classes have begun to shift from muscle isolation exercises to functional exercises that are sport-specific and may improve participants' ability to perform activities of daily living.

Benefits

Some potential participants may avoid group strength training due to misconceptions about the effects of regular strength training. They may not understand the important role strength training plays in losing or maintaining body weight. Also, in some cases, women may believe that strength training will create bulky muscles. To keep exercise motivation high, communicate the benefits with participants before, during, and after class. For example, explain that strength training improves physical working capacity and appearance, metabolic function, and injury risk. Use positive statements to sell the benefits of strength training.

To emphasize physical working capacity, relate how exercises will help with real-life tasks that require strength.

"This exercise will help you lift boxes onto a high shelf."

"This exercise will help you carry your kids upstairs."

When focusing on physical appearance and metabolic functioning, explain how the exercises will help in maintaining or reducing body weight.

"These exercises help us burn more fat, even when we are sleeping."

"These exercises will help us burn all those extra calories we consumed over the holidays."

To explain the reduced injury risk, relate how the exercises help prevent injury or muscular imbalances.

"This exercise helps us with our posture."

"This exercise helps prevent lower-back pain."

An effective strength-training program will provide the following physiological improvements:

- Increased muscle fiber size
- Increased muscle contractile strength
- Increased tendon tensile strength
- Increased bone strength
- Increased ligament tensile strength

Kinesiology

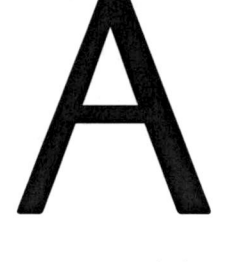basic understanding of kinesiology will enable you to elect the right exercise to target specific muscle groups, offer modifications, and manage risk.

If, for example, during side deltoid raises, the participant becomes fatigued and begins to "throw" or jerk the weights, you can make the following analysis:

1. The targeted muscle group is not being effectively strengthened, because the legs and torso are being used to initiate the lifting motion. The initial burst of movement carries the weight through the rest of the motion with only slight use of the deltoids.

2. One possible modification is to bend the elbows 90 degrees to reduce the effective resistance and make the participant more aware of form. If there is no improvement in form, reduce the resistance.

3. The snapping motion used to initiate the movement compromises the stability of the shoulder joint. Lifting more slowly and with control allows the rotator cuff muscle group to stabilize the shoulder joint more effectively.

Line of Gravity

With dumbbells and weighted bars, the effectiveness of any given exercise is largely dependent on whether the movement falls within the line of gravity. For example, consider a single-arm triceps kick-back exercise. A common error during this exercise is to allow the weight to swing past 90 degrees to 45 degrees of elbow flexion.

The starting, or resting, position of the exercise is with the upper arm parallel to the floor and the lower arm perpendicular to the floor so that the elbow is flexed 90 degrees. The line of gravity is a straight line from the ceiling to the floor and is in the same direction as the lower arm. During elbow **extension,** the triceps work to lift the weight against gravity. The triceps also work as the weight is lowered back toward the resting position. As the arm moves past 90 degrees of elbow flexion, it is the biceps that are working to lift the weights against gravity (Figure 2.1).

Any exercise can be analyzed to determine when the movement falls within the line of gravity.

Figure 2.1
Line of gravity. The single-arm triceps kick-back is a good example of the importance of understanding of how the line of gravity affects a movement.

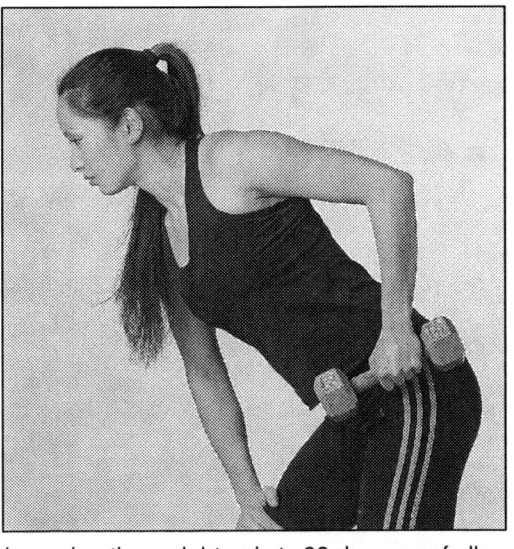

Lowering the weight only to 90 degrees of elbow flexion ensures that the triceps are working throughout the exercise.

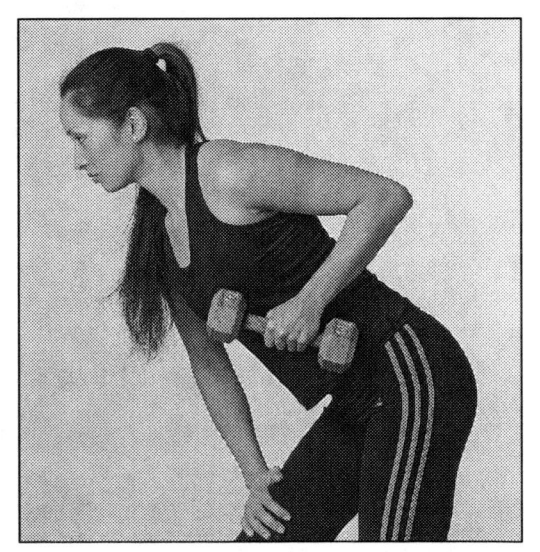

Moving to 45 degrees of elbow flexion shifts the workload to the biceps.

Exercise Analysis

Exercise #1: Standing chest fly with dumbbells

Targeted muscle group: Chest

Action: The start position is with the arms in 90 degrees of shoulder abduction from the sides of the body (Figure 2.2a). The action is 90 degrees of horizontal shoulder adduction in the transverse plane followed by 90 degrees of horizontal shoulder abduction in the transverse plane (Figure 2.2b).

Analysis: Ineffective, because the action of the exercise does not fall within the line of gravity.

The chest group is targeted, but the deltoids are the primary muscle group for this exercise. Because the deltoids create a force equal to the gravitational force, the weights remain in the transverse plane.

Solution: Perform the chest fly from a supine position so the exercise falls within the line of gravity, or substitute elastic resistance for the dumbbells so that the exercise falls within the line of resistance created by the elastic resistance (Figure 2.2c).

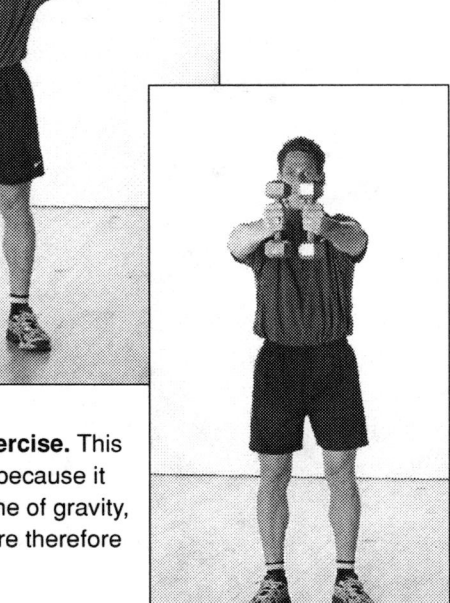

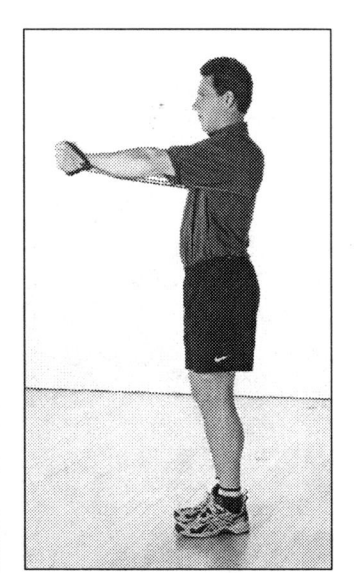

Figures 2.2a&b
Ineffective chest fly exercise. This movement is ineffective because it does not fall within the line of gravity, and the chest muscles are therefore not being targeted.

Figure 2.2c
An appropriate modification. Replacing the dumbbells with elastic resistance negates the importance of the line of gravity and the chest muscles are now effectively targeted.

Exercise #2: Standing biceps curls with dumbbells

Targeted muscle group: Biceps

Action: The start position is with the arms extended down the sides of the body. The action is 180 degrees of elbow flexion in the sagittal plane followed by 180 degrees of elbow extension in the sagittal plane.

Analysis: Good. The exercise falls within the line of gravity during most of the movement. The weight and gravity are constant forces, but the amount of force necessary to move the weight changes as the elbow flexes and extends. The force is determined by the lever arm, the distance from the elbow joint (the fulcrum) to the weight. The force required to move the weight increases proportionately as the **lever** arm increases (i.e., the muscle force required to lift the weight increases as the horizontal distance from the elbow joint to the weight increases). At the extremes of the exercise (the first and last 15 degrees of the exercise), the biceps are working dramatically less than at 90 degrees (Figure 2.3).

Modification: Modify the exercise to a single-arm curl with the other arm adding manual resistance near the wrist between the hand and the elbow.

Figure 2.3
Standing biceps curl

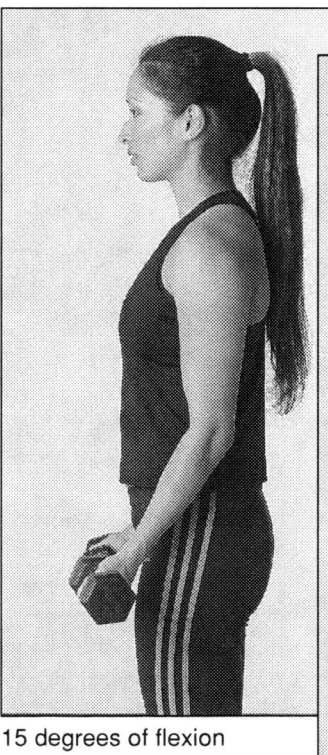
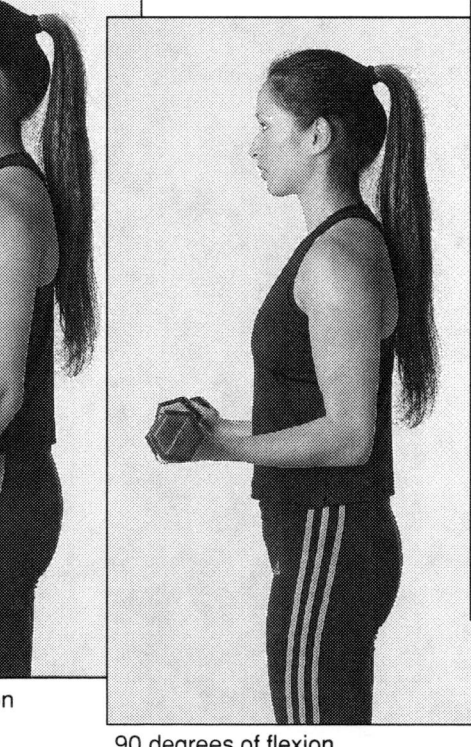
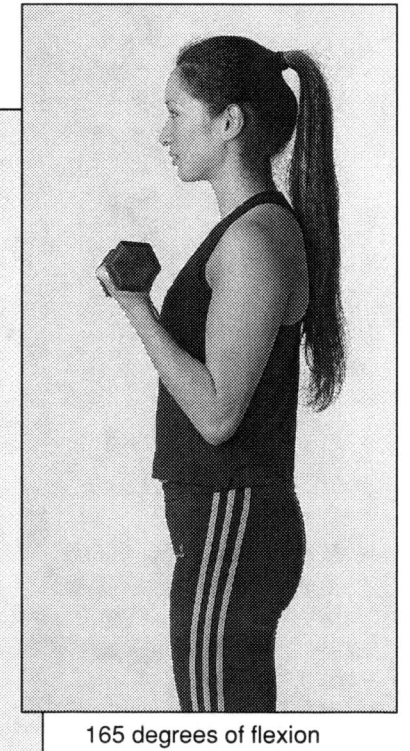

165 degrees of flexion

15 degrees of flexion

90 degrees of flexion

Types of Contractions

There are three types of muscular contractions utilized in any strength-training program.

Isometric

During an **isometric** contraction there is no joint movement. For example, an isometric chest exercise can be performed by placing the palms of the hands together about one foot away from the chest. Next, each hand exerts an equal and opposite force resulting in a muscular contraction without any motion.

Concentric

During a **concentric** contraction there is a shortening of the muscle length (e.g., the up phase of the biceps curl, in which the biceps muscle group shortens as the elbow joint flexes).

Eccentric

During an **eccentric** contraction the length of the muscle increases (e.g., the down phase of the biceps curl, in which the biceps muscle group lengthens as the elbow joint extends).

Exercise Analysis

The following questions will guide you in analyzing and designing effective exercises.

1. What movements occur at each joint?
2. Is the movement slow or fast?
3. Is the motion occurring against gravity or in the same direction? Against resistance or not?
4. What muscles are causing the joint movement?
5. Is the contraction concentric, eccentric, or isometric?
6. Which muscles are movers and which are stabilizers?
7. Does the movement achieve the stated goal of the exercise?
8. Does the exercise train the primary function of the muscle?
9. Does the movement compromise the safety of other body parts? Are nonmoving joints stabilized adequately in neutral?
10. How can the exercise be adapted to meet the specific needs of the client (i.e., made more or less difficult)?

Equipment

There is a variety of equipment that can be used to modify basic strength-training exercises. The equipment falls into three categories.

1. Dynamic constant resistance equipment, which includes weighted bars, dumbbells, and any other equipment in which the resistance stays constant.

2. Dynamic variable resistance equipment, which includes bands, tubes, and other elastic equipment.

3. Exercise props, which include mats, benches, steps, stability balls, or any other equipment that is used during the exercise.

Exercise mats can be used for more than comfort. Mats that can be folded or rolled can be used as an incline bench during chest flys, or to increase recruitment of stabilizers during a push-up (Figure 2.4).

Constant vs. Variable Exercise Equipment

There are three major differences between constant and variable exercise equipment: elastic properties, line of gravity, and degree of stress on the joints.

Elastic properties

The elastic nature of the elastic resistance causes the intensity to increase as the band lengthens. Conversely, the weight of dumbbells stays constant through the entire range of motion.

Line of gravity

To effectively perform strength-training exercises with dumbbells, the weight must be lifted and lowered within the line of gravity. Variable exercise equipment does not depend on the line of gravity, but rather the line of resistance.

Figure 2.4
Exercise mats can be used for more than comfort.

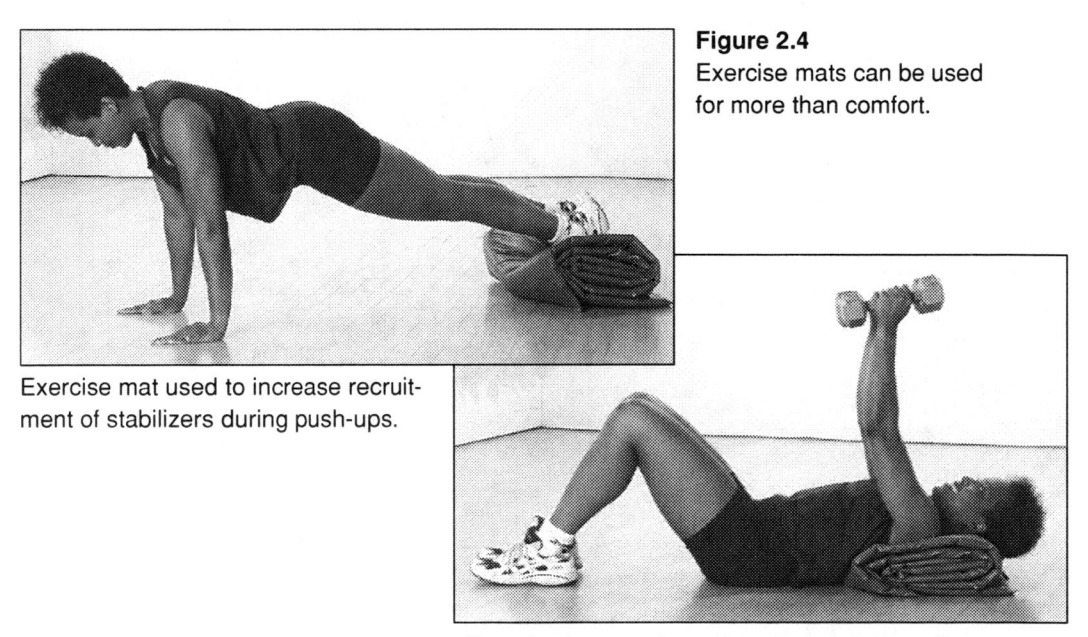

Exercise mat used to increase recruitment of stabilizers during push-ups.

Exercise mat used as a bench during chest flies.

For example, to work external rotation of the shoulder joint, the participant must lie on his or her side to effectively utilize the line of gravity. With a band, the exercise can be performed while standing. If the band is held on the opposite hip, the line of resistance created by the angle of the band is within the line of movement.

Stress on joints

Because of the properties of elastic resistance, the stress placed on the joint tends to be different than that caused by weights. During an overhead triceps extension, starting at 90 degrees of elbow flexion, the force on the elbow joint is vastly different during the movement. With elastic resistance, there is less force on the elbow joint at the beginning of the movement compared to greater forces on the elbow joint at the end of the movement. Conversely, the force on the elbow joint is greater at the beginning of the movement compared to the end of the movement when using weights.

General Strength-training Guidelines

Exercise Selection

Select at least one exercise for each major muscle group to ensure comprehensive muscle development. Training only a few muscle groups leads to muscular imbalance and may increase the risk of injury. Therefore, design a strength-training program that addresses muscle balance and incorporates exercises for areas that typically receive less attention.

Exercise Sequence

When developing a circuit of strength exercises, proceed from the larger muscle groups of the legs to the smaller muscle groups of the torso, arms, and neck. In this way, the most demanding exercises are performed when participants are least fatigued. Also, perform exercises that are more complex and neurologically challenging at the beginning of a circuit, and do not excessively fatigue the core prior to performing these exercises, as this increases the risk of injury.

Exercise Speed

Lift slowly to work the muscle through the entire range of motion. Lifting quickly places excessive stress on the muscles, tendons, and ligaments during the initiation of the movement and increases the risk of injury. The recommended speed is one or two seconds for the concentric muscle action followed by three to four seconds for the eccentric muscle action.

Exercise Sets

An exercise set is usually defined as a number of successive repetitions performed without resting. Although the greatest strength gains are derived from multiple sets and repetitions, the number of sets is a matter of personal preference and time considerations. An advantage of multiple-set strength training is that it allows participants to repeat exercises

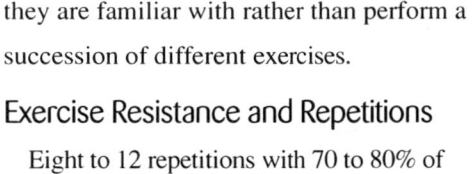

they are familiar with rather than perform a succession of different exercises.

Exercise Resistance and Repetitions

Eight to 12 repetitions with 70 to 80% of maximum resistance is optimal for safe and effective strength development. When exercises are performed in a slow and controlled manner, this requires about 50 to 60 seconds of high-intensity (anaerobic) muscle effort.

Exercise Range

Perform each exercise through a full range of motion, with an emphasis on the fully contracted position. A full range of motion promotes joint flexibility. Only reduce the range of motion when the full range of motion compromises joint stability or if joint pain occurs.

Exercise Progression

When a participant can easily perform 12 or more repetitions with good form, it is time to increase the workload by 5% or less. Limitations in equipment often make it seem impossible to increase the workload. By using both weights and elastic resistance or by adding manual resistance, workloads can be increased even with only light resistance equipment (Figure 2.5).

Exercise Frequency

Because the muscle rebuilding process typically requires 48 hours, strength workouts that exercise the same muscle group should be scheduled every other day to allow full recovery.

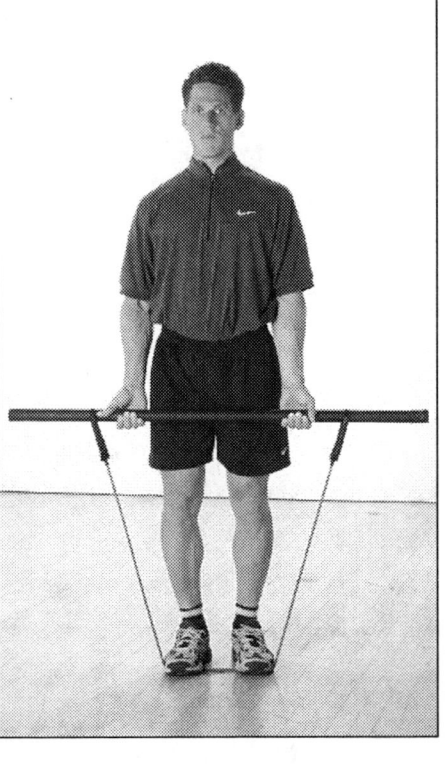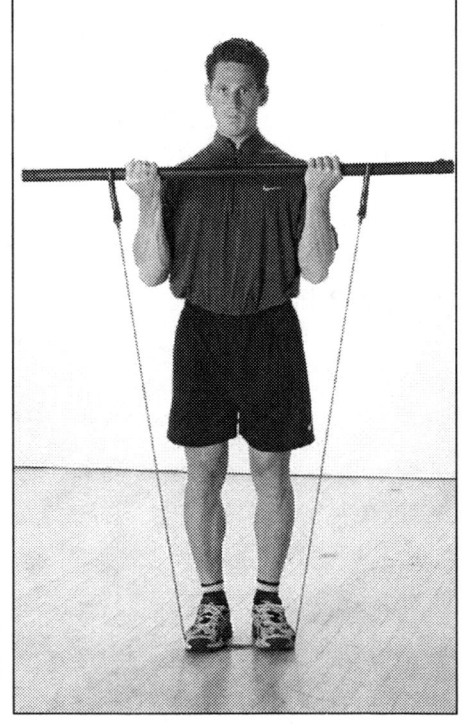

Figure 2.5 Combine weights and elastic resistance to increase intensity.

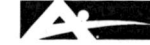

Group Strength Training Techniques

CHAPTER THREE

The following exercises are grouped by body part, each with a table listing exercises by starting position and equipment. The tables will assist in creating smooth transitions between exercises. Remember to only alter one aspect (i.e., equipment or position) during each transition.

Common strength-training errors

Watch for the following flaws in technique, which are common to many strength-training exercises.

Error: Increasing the natural arch in the lower back
Correction: Slightly engage the abdominals to maintain neutral spine and provide low-back support.

Error: Using the legs and momentum to perform a lift; rocking or jerking during the exercise; performing the movement too quickly
Correction: Begin the movement slowly and with control; pause at the top and bottom of each repetition.

Error: Forward neck posture
Correction: Keep the neck in neutral position and in alignment with the spine.

Chest

Muscles involved: Pectoralis major, anterior and middle deltoid, triceps

Strength-training techniques for the chest:

1. A narrow grip during the exercise increases the involvement of the triceps. Conversely, widening the grip decreases the involvement of the triceps.

2. When performing chest flys, keep the palms facing each other and allow a slight flexion in the elbows to reduce the stress on the shoulder joint.

3. During push-ups and chest flys, horizontal abduction beyond 90 degrees places excessive stress on the shoulder joint.

Table 3.1
Exercises for the Chest

Position	Resistance	Exercises
Standing	Elastic	Chest press (with partner)
		Chest fly
Standing	Bodyweight	Wall push-up
Prone	Bodyweight	Push-up
		Triceps push-up
Supine	Weights	Chest press (on bench)
		Chest fly (on bench)
Supine	Elastic	Chest press
		Chest fly (on bench)

Push-up

Targeted muscles: Pectoralis major, anterior deltoids, triceps

Starting position: Begin on the floor with the hands slightly wider than shoulder-width apart. Place toes or knees onto floor, depending on the level of resistance needed. Keep the back straight and torso supported by engaging the abdominals throughout the exercise (Figure 3.1).

Action: Press the body up to the point just prior to locked elbows (Figure 3.2). Pause, then lower until elbows are at approximately a 90-degree angle.

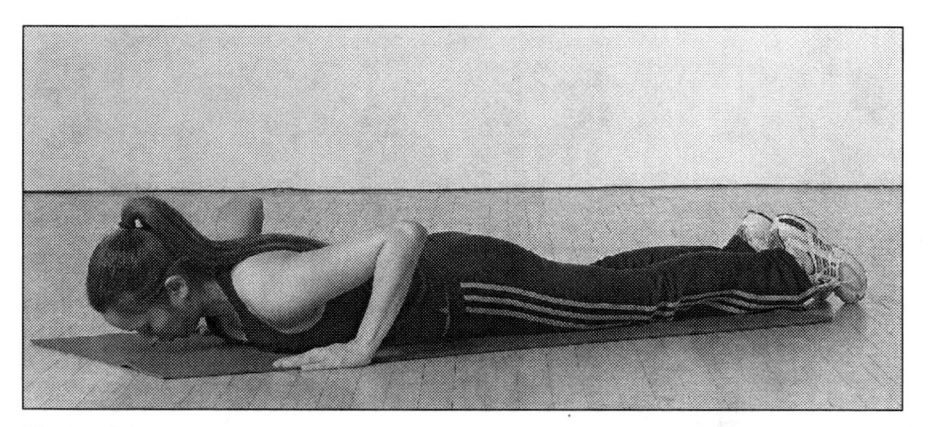

Figure 3.1
Push-up; starting position

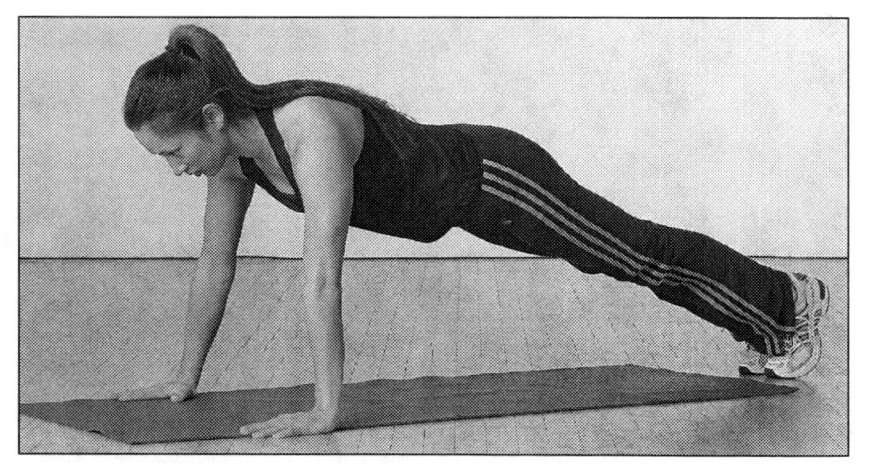

Figure 3.2
Push-up; action

Variations:

• For deconditioned participants: wall push-
  ups (Figure 3.3)

• Incline: hands on a bench or step (Figure 3.4)

• Decline: feet on a bench or exercise ball
  (Figure 3.5)

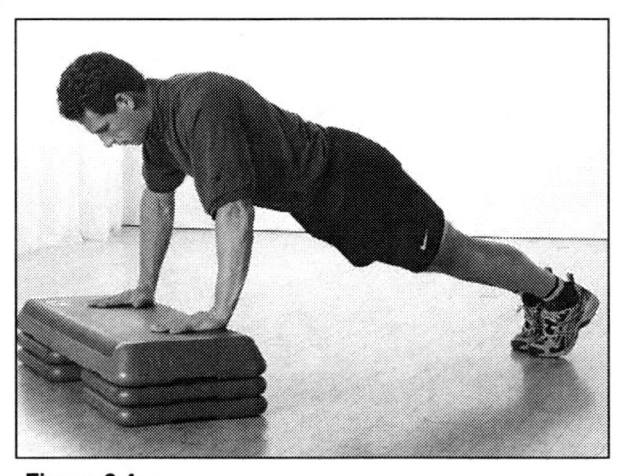

Figure 3.4
Push-up variation;
Use a bench to create an incline.

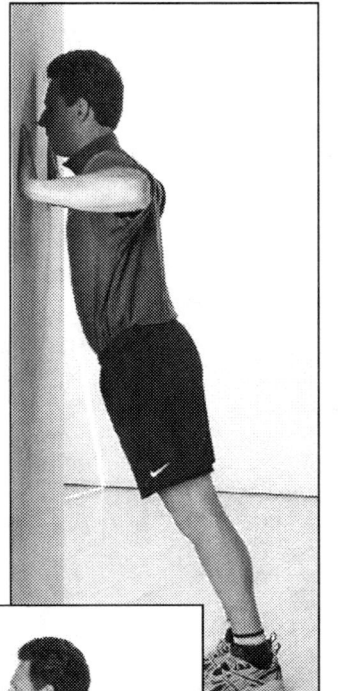

Figure 3.3
Wall
push-up

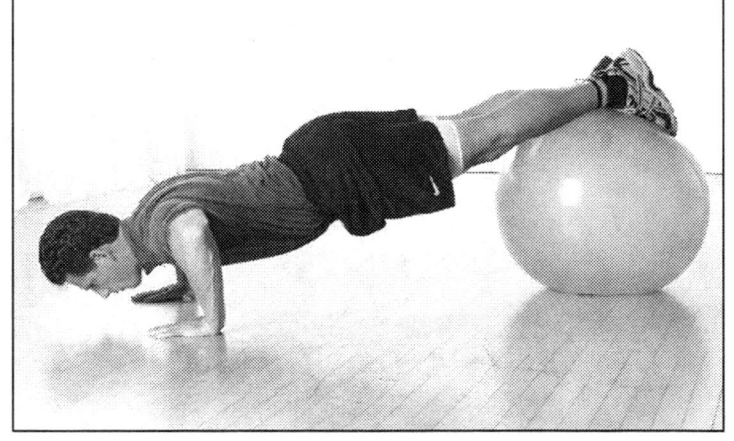

Figure 3.5
Push-up variation;
Use a stability ball to create a decline.

• Keeping the elbows close to the body emphasizes the anterior deltoid and triceps (Figure 3.6).

Equipment variation:

• Chest press with elastic resistance (Figure 3.7).

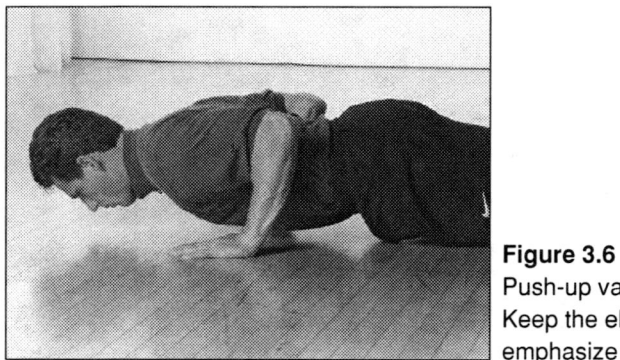

Figure 3.6
Push-up variation;
Keep the elbows close to the body to emphasize the anterior deltoid and triceps.

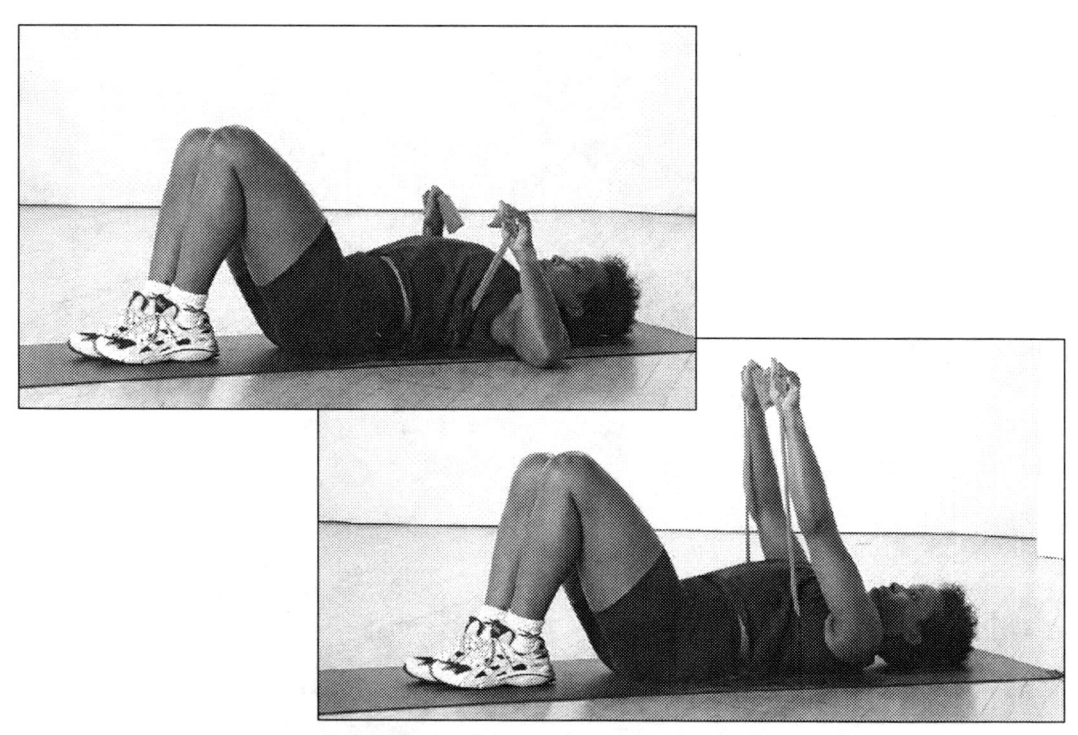

Figure 3.7
Push-up variation;
When working with clients with carpal tunnel syndrome or other sources of wrist pain, use elastic resistance to perform chest presses as an alternative to push-ups.

Supine Chest Fly

Targeted muscles: Pectoralis major, anterior deltoids

Starting position: Begin supine on the floor or bench with bent knees. Start with arms extended directly above your shoulders with your elbows slightly bent. Lower weights to about 90 degrees of shoulder abduction or to a comfortable stretch in the pectorals (Figure 3.8).

Action: Adduct the arms to the point above the shoulder joints (Figure 3.9). Pause, then slowly lower the arms to the starting position.

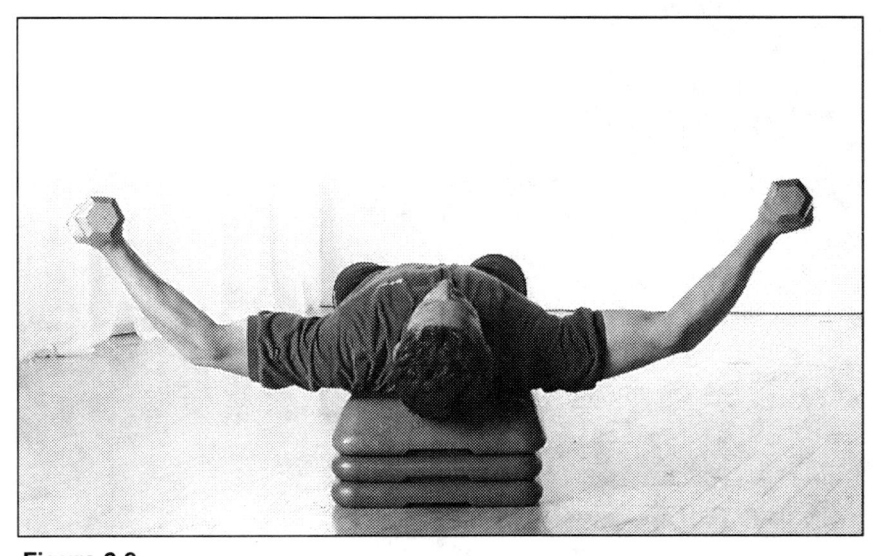

Figure 3.8
Supine chest fly; starting position

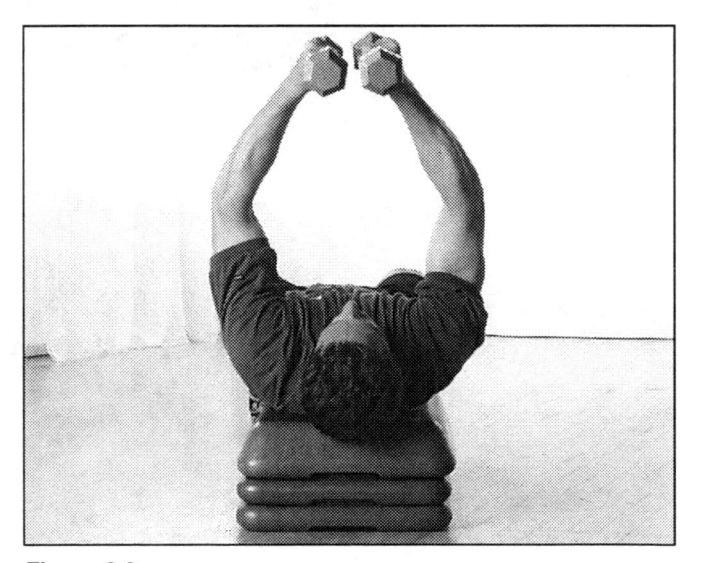

Figure 3.9
Supine chest fly; action

Common error:

Error: Lowering the arms too quickly and going past the comfortable starting position

Correction: Emphasize lowering the weights slowly and not letting the hands move out of peripheral vision.

Variation:

• Incline or decline with a bench

Equipment variation:

• Elastic resistance in the standing or supine position with resistance placed behind the back (Figure 3.10)

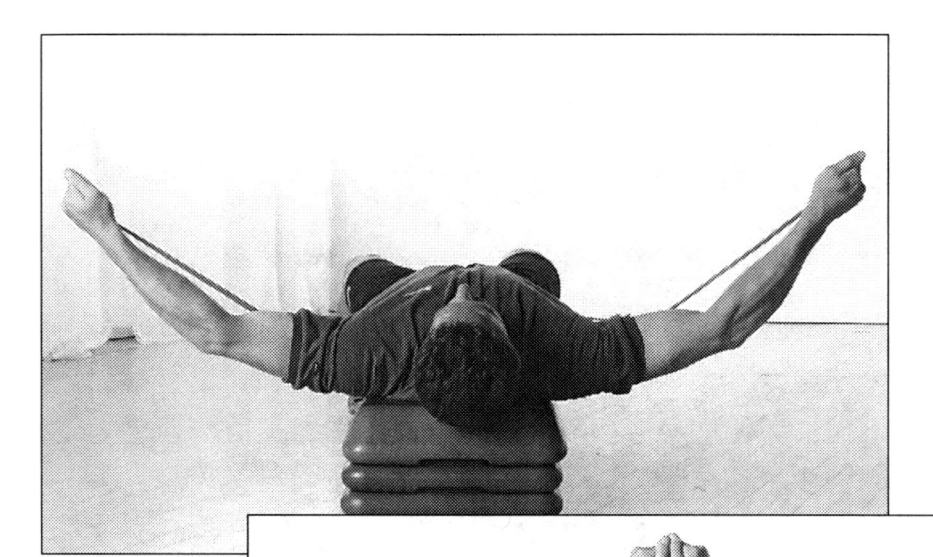

Figure 3.10
Supine chest fly variation; elastic resistance

Chest Press

Targeted muscles: Pectoralis major, anterior deltoids, triceps

Starting position: Begin supine on the floor or bench with bent knees. Hold dumbbells or bar with arms extended directly over the shoulders with elbows slightly bent. With straight wrists, lower weights by bending the elbows to a point of comfortable stretch for the chest muscles (Figure 3.11).

Action: Press the weight up to a point just before full elbow extension (Figure 3.12) Pause, then slowly lower weight to the starting position.

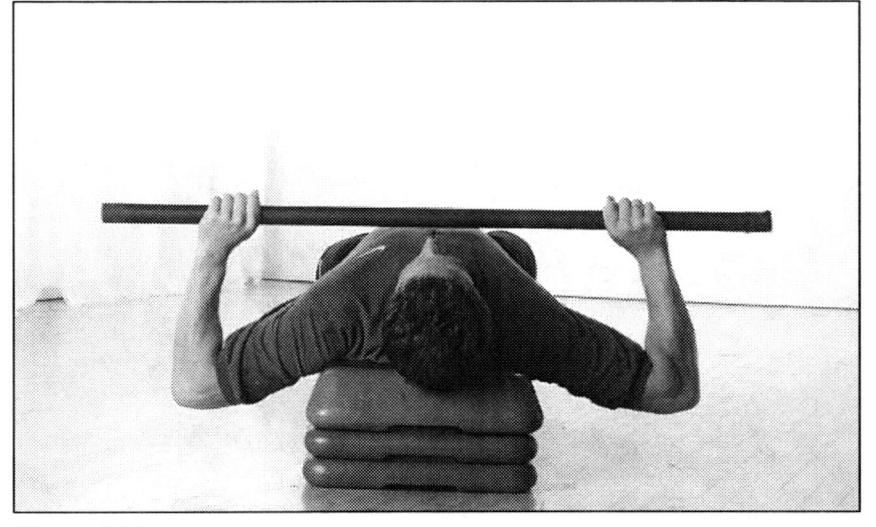

Figure 3.11
Chest press; starting position

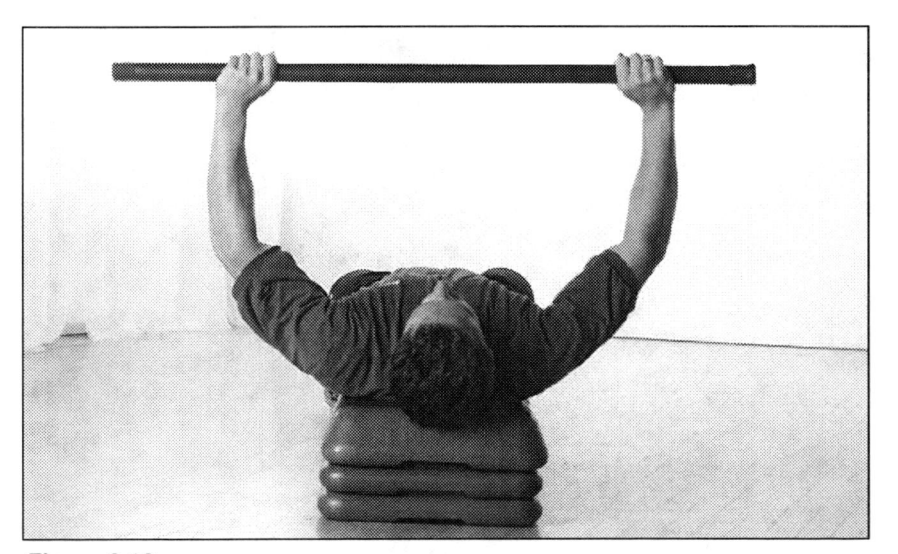

Figure 3.12
Chest press; action

Common errors:

Error: Bent wrists (forward or backward)

Correction: Keep weight stacked over the wrist with a light grip.

Error: Lowering the arms too quickly and going past the comfortable starting position

Correction: Emphasize lowering the weights slowly and not letting the hands go below the peripheral vision.

Variation:

• Elbows close to the body emphasizes more anterior deltoid and triceps

Equipment variations:

• Have a partner hold elastic resistance around the back (Figure 3.13).

• Use a bench to create incline or decline modification.

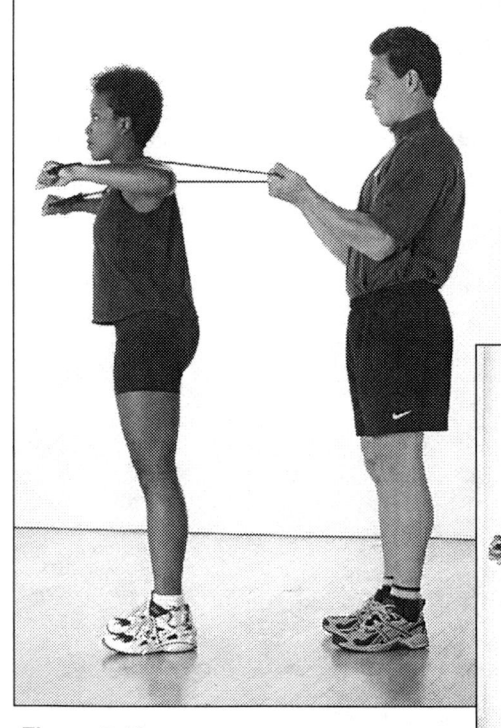

Figure 3.13
Chest press variation; elastic resistance with a partner

Back

Muscles involved: Latissimus dorsi, trapezius, rhomboids, teres major, levator scapula

Strength-training techniques for the back:

1. A narrow grip during the exercise increases the involvement of the biceps. Conversely, widening the grip decreases the involvement of the biceps.

2. During forward flexion, look for opportunities to provide additional support to the spine. Offer a single-arm modification to allow the opposite arm to help support the spine. Sustained unsupported forward flexion can lead to lower-back pain if the abdominals are not engaged or if the lumbar spine flexes. Maintaining the natural lumbar curve, and therefore a neutral spine, is important during all exercises.

3. During rowing motion, keep the torso from rotating to isolate the primary muscle group.

4. During upright rows, minimize inward rotation of the shoulder by raising the upper arms only to shoulder height. The starting point is with the arms close to the body. During the concentric muscle action, move the hands forward on a 15-degree angle to reduce the stress on the shoulder.

5. During lat pull-down exercises, bring the hands down in front of the body rather than behind the neck to reduce the stress on the shoulder joint and neck.

Table 3.2
Exercises for the Back

Position	Resistance	Exercises
Standing	Weights	Bent-over row
		Single-arm row
		Shoulder shrug
		Upright row
		Scapular retraction
Standing	Elastic	Shoulder shrug
		Single-arm lat pull-down
		Upright row
Seated	Elastic	Seated row
All-fours	Weights	Scapular retraction (on bench)

Bent-over Row

Targeted muscles: Latissimus dorsi, teres major, posterior deltoid, trapezius, rhomboids, biceps

Starting position: Standing, begin with feet shoulder-width apart, bend the knees, and flex forward at the hips. Tilt the pelvis slightly forward, engage the abdominals, and extend the upper spine to add support to the spine. Hold the weight or bar beneath the shoulders with hands about shoulder-width apart (Figure 3.14).

Action: Flex the elbows and lift the hands toward the sides of the body (Figure 3.15). Pause, then slowly lower the hands to the starting position.

Common error:

Error: Allowing the shoulders to roll forward

Correction: Keep the shoulders stationary.

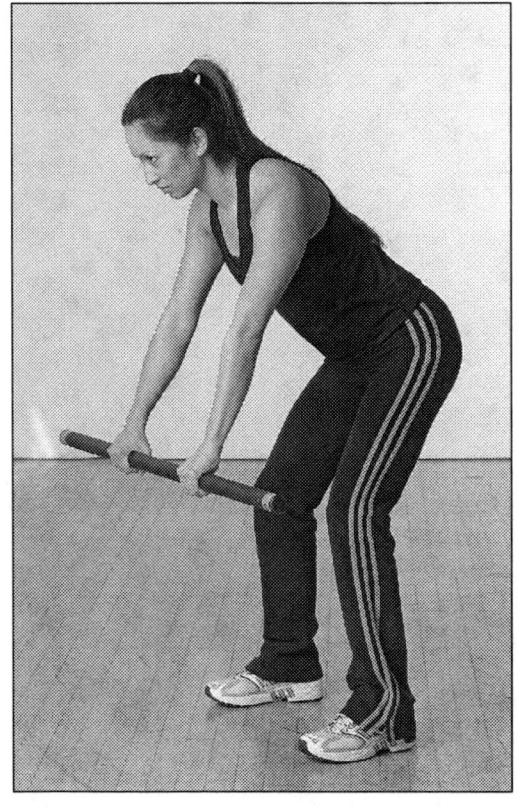

Figure 3.14
Bent-over row; starting position

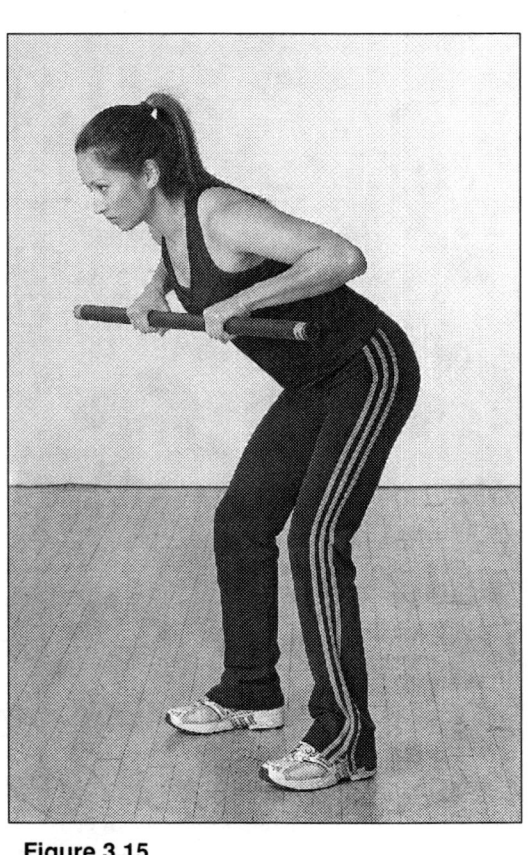

Figure 3.15
Bent-over row; action

Variation:

• Single-arm row with the legs in a staggered position and one hand on the front thigh for support, with the arm rotated inward so the fingers are toward the inner thigh (Figure 3.16)

Equipment variations:

• Lying face down on an incline bench
• One arm and knee on a bench for support

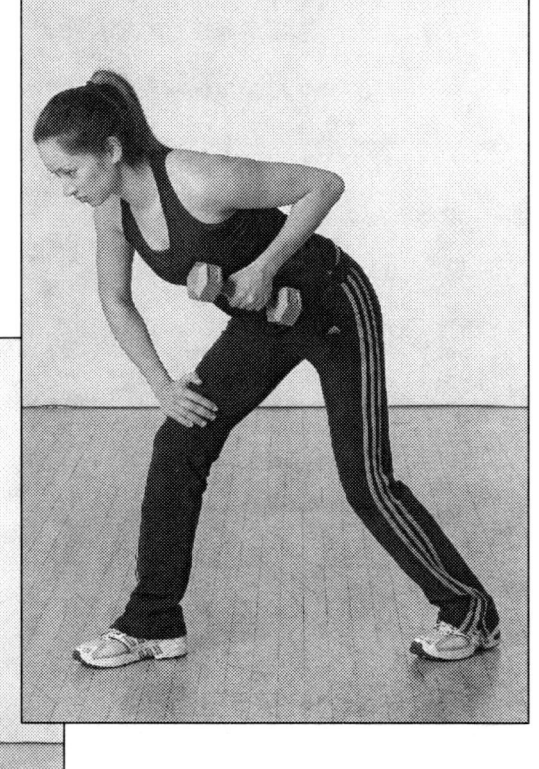

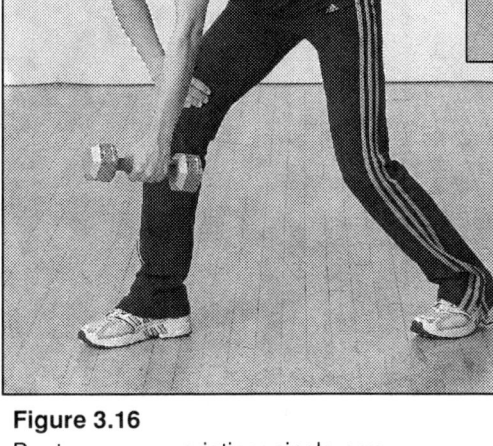

Figure 3.16
Bent-over row variation; single-arm

Shoulder Shrug

Targeted muscles: Trapezius, rhomboids, levator scapula

Starting position: Stand erect with dumbbells held at the sides of the body (Figure 3.17).

Action: Lift the shoulders toward the head by elevating the shoulder girdle, and slightly retract the scapulae to rotate the shoulders back (Figure 3.18). Pause, then return to the starting position.

Common errors:

Error: Rocking or using the legs to initiate the exercise

Correction: Maintain slightly bent knees.

Error: Bending the elbows

Correction: Relax the upper arms and lift using the upper back.

Error: Rounding the shoulders forward while elevating them

Correction: Remain open through the anterior shoulders and chest by slightly retracting the scapulae.

Variation:

• Perform one shoulder at a time.

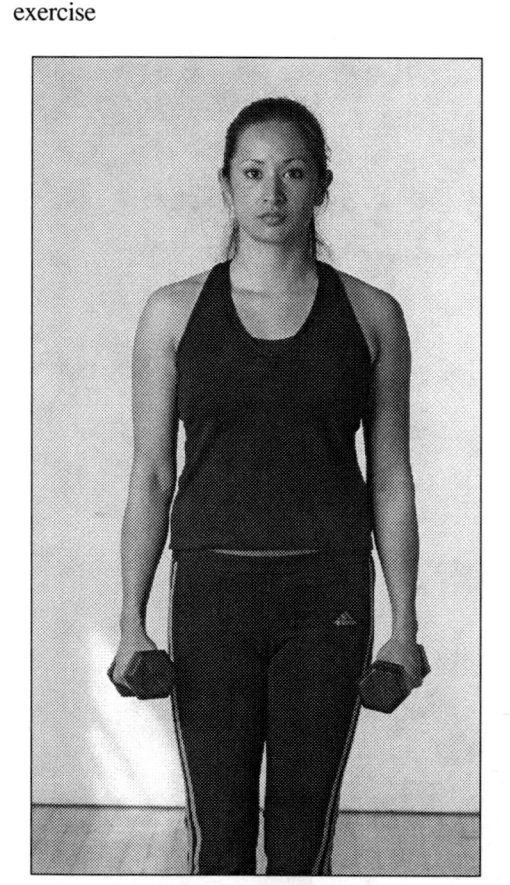

Figure 3.17
Shoulder shrug; starting position

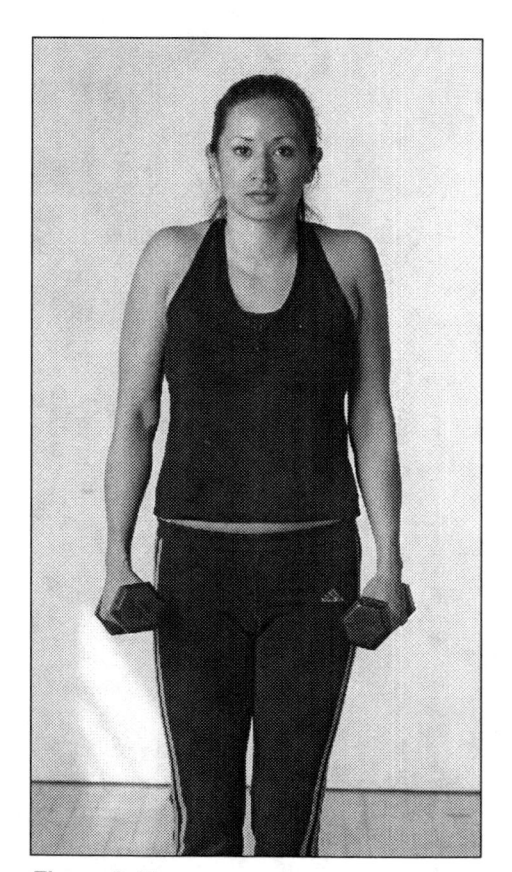

Figure 3.18
Shoulder shrug; action

Equipment variation:

• Elastic resistance; perform in a staggered or
standing position with band anchored under the
feet (Figure 3.19)

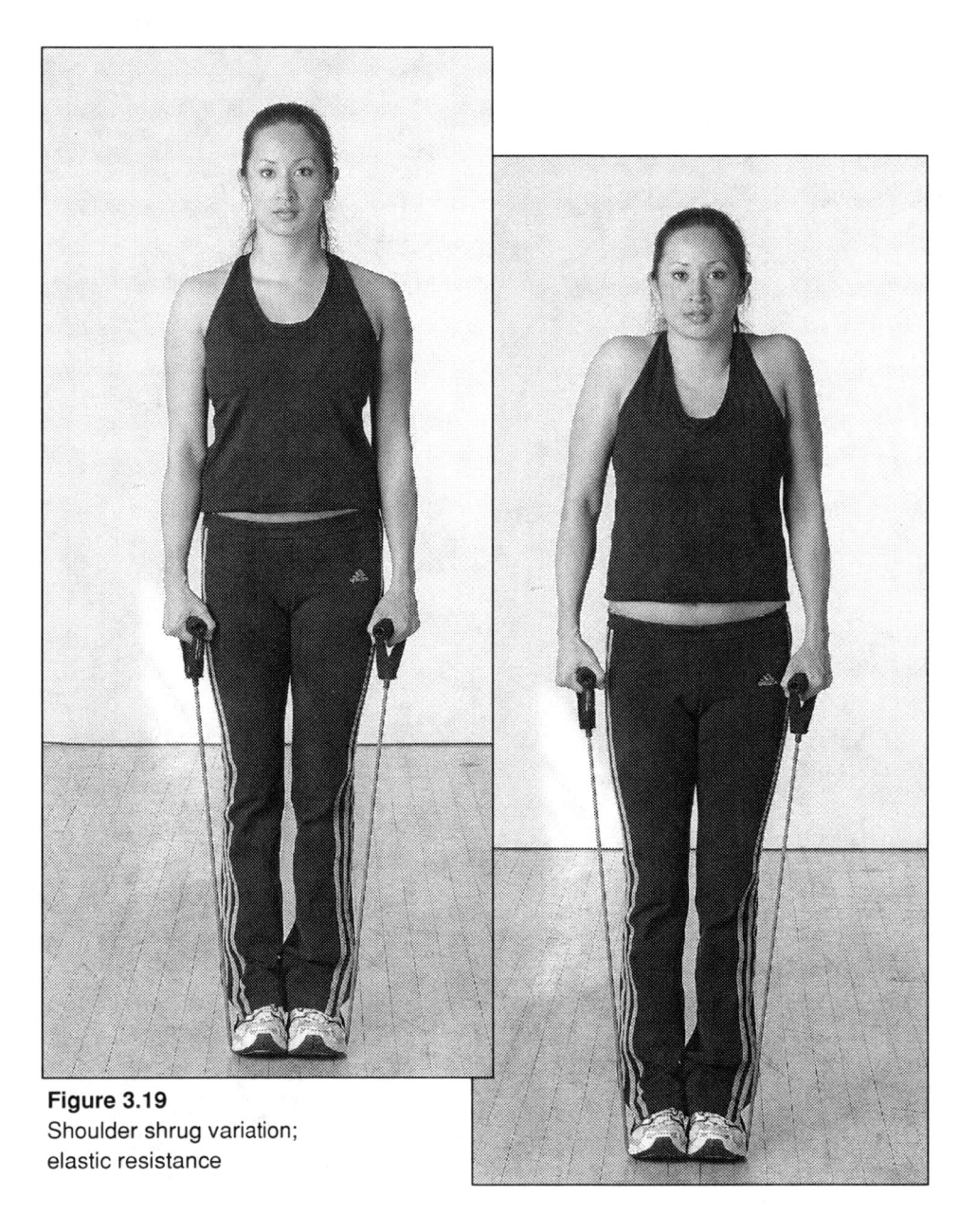

Figure 3.19
Shoulder shrug variation;
elastic resistance

Upright Row

Targeted muscles: Deltoids, trapezius

Starting position: Begin with dumbbells held in front of the body (Figure 3.20).

Action: Stabilize the shoulder girdle by slightly retracting and depressing the scapulae (Figure 3.21). Lead with the elbows and raise the arms until the upper arms are shoulder height (keep dumbbells close to the body throughout) (Figure 3.22). Pause, then slowly return to the starting position.

Common error:

Error: Lifting the elbows too high

Correction: Keep the elbows at or below shoulder height.

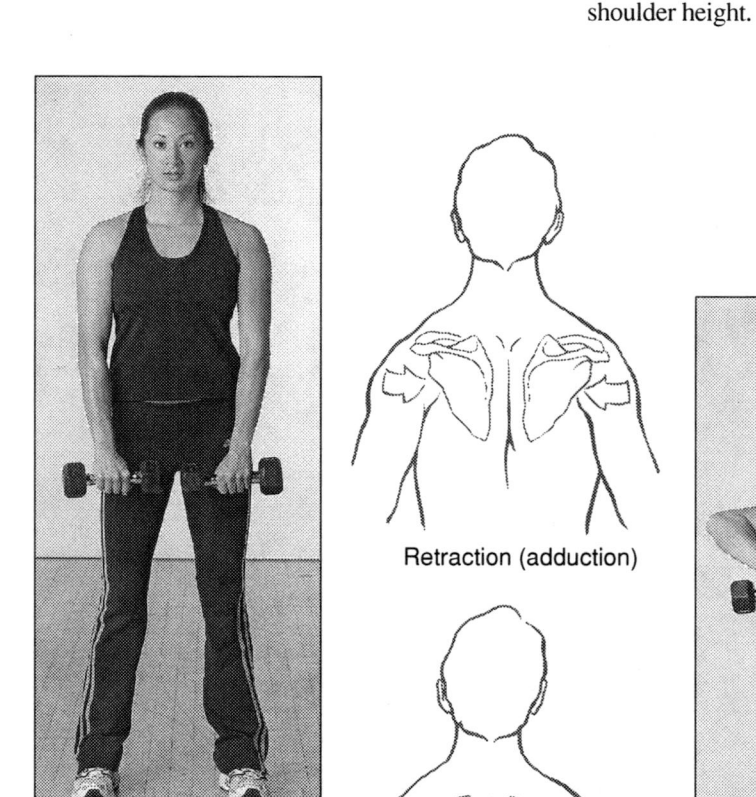

Retraction (adduction)

Depression

Figure 3.21
Scapular movements; stabilizing the shoulder girdle

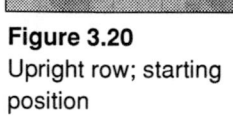

Figure 3.20
Upright row; starting position

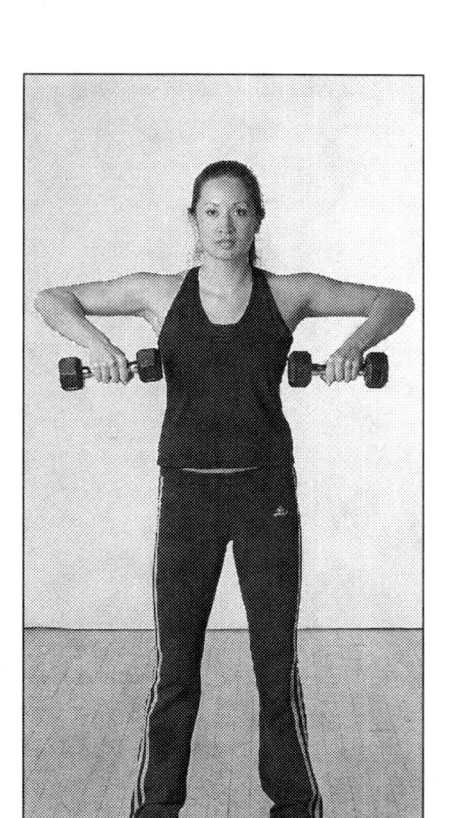

Figure 3.22
Upright row; action

Variation:

• One arm at a time; during the lift, move the hands forward away from the body to reduce the stress on the shoulder joints.

Equipment variation:

• Elastic resistance; can be performed in standing or staggered position with the band anchored below the feet (Figure 3.23)

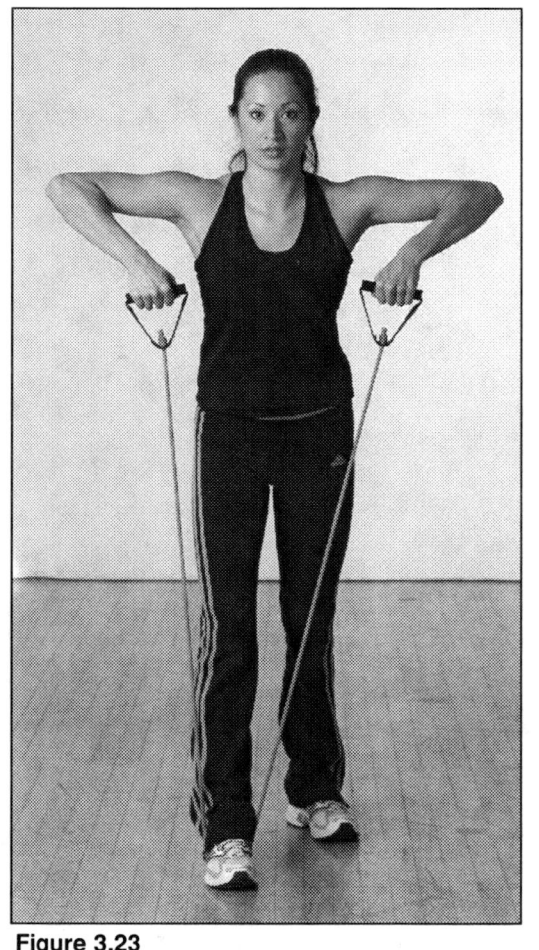

Figure 3.23
Upright row variation; elastic resistance

Single-arm Lat Pull-down

Targeted muscle: Latissimus dorsi, teres major, lower trapezius, posterior deltoid

Starting position: Begin with both hands overhead holding an elastic resistance band; maintain neutral wrists and soft joints. Engage the abdominals, bend the knees slightly, and position the feet about shoulder-width apart (Figure 3.24).

Action: Pull downward to the side with one arm, adducting at the shoulder until the upper arm is next to the torso (Figure 3.25). Pause, then return slowly to the starting position.

Keep arms slightly in front of the face to protect the back and shoulders.

Common errors:

Error: Flexing the wrist

Correction: Keep the hand stacked over the top of the wrist.

Error: Allowing the arms to drift back behind the neck

Correction: Keep the hands in peripheral vision at all times.

Variation:

• Bend the non-working elbow to decrease the resistance and reduce the stress on the shoulder joint.

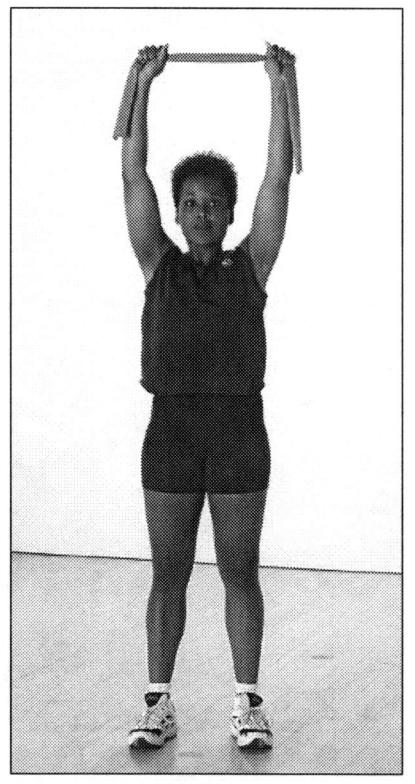

Figure 3.24
Single-arm lat pull-down using elastic resistance; starting position

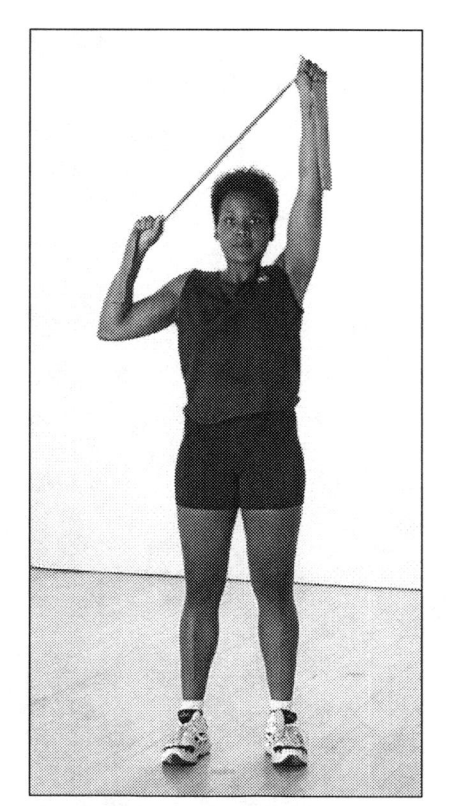

Figure 3.25
Single-arm lat pull-down using elastic resistance; action

Scapular Retraction

Targeted muscles: Rhomboids, trapezius

Starting position: Begin with feet about shoulder-width apart and the pelvis tilted slightly forward; engage the abdominals to help maintain neutral spine. Flex forward and hold dumbbells extended down away from the body (Figure 3.26).

Action: Adduct shoulder blades together (Figure 3.27). Pause, then slowly return to the starting position.

Common error:

Error: Bending the elbows

Correction: Relax the upper arms and lift using the upper back.

Variation:

• Single arm

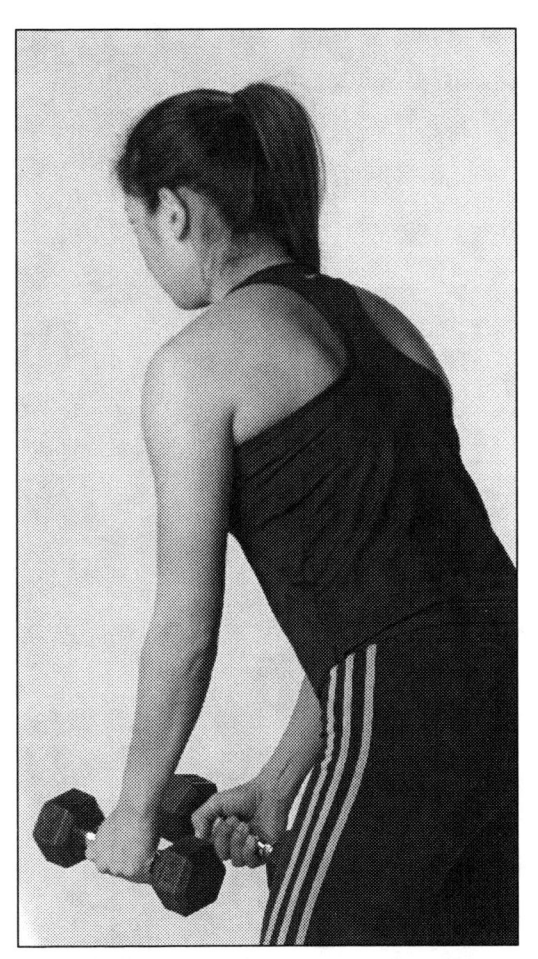

Figure 3.26
Scapular retraction; starting position

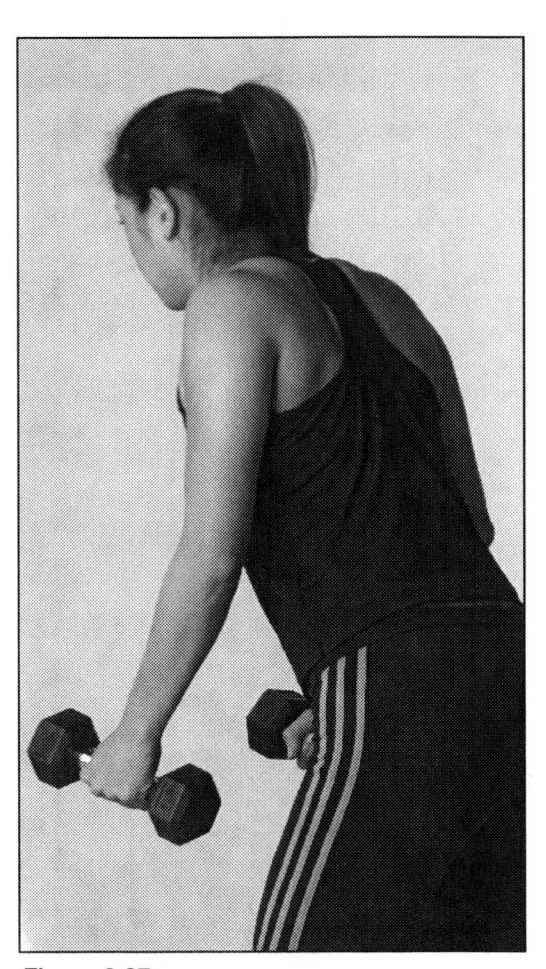

Figure 3.27
Scapular retraction; action

Equipment variations:

• Prone on a bench or with one arm and both

 knees on the bench (Figure 3.28)

• Elastic resistance anchored at the feet

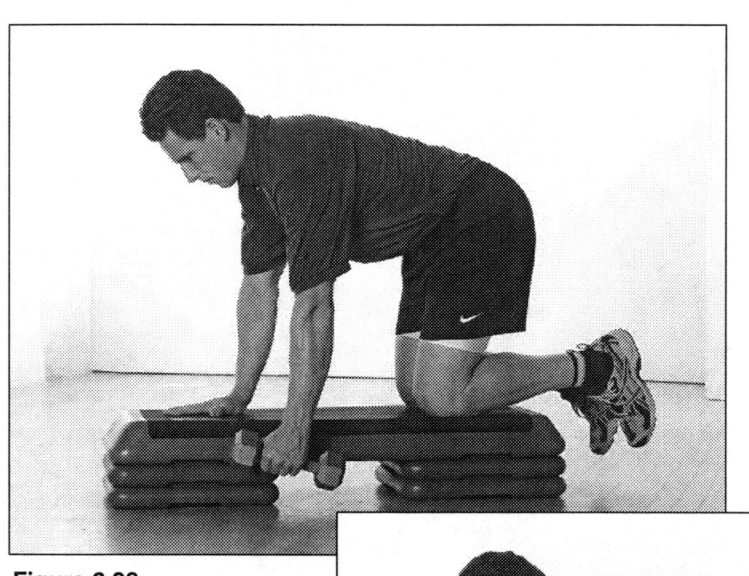

Figure 3.28
Scapular retraction
variation; single-arm with
one hand and both knees
on a bench

Seated Row

Targeted muscles: Rhomboids, latissimus dorsi, teres major, trapezius

Starting position: Sit with the legs extended in front, with the knees bent if necessary to reach the feet. Begin by securing a band around your feet (Figure 3.29).

Figure 3.29
Securing the elastic band to the feet.

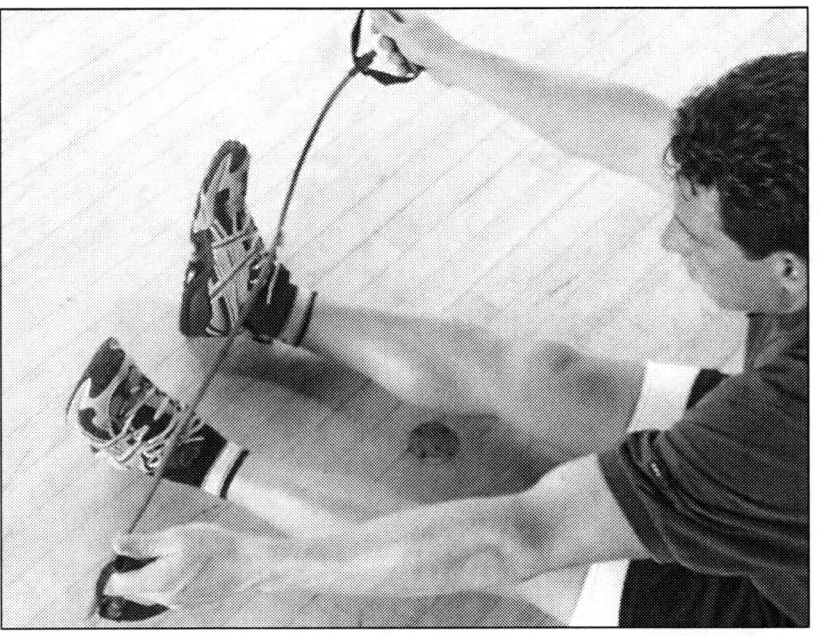

Place elastic band across the top of the shoes, over the shoelaces.

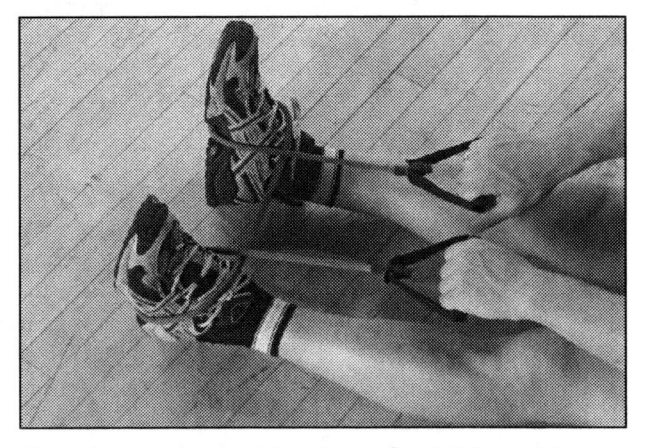

Wrap the band around the shoes. Start at the outside of the shoes and wrap toward the bottom of shoes. Draw the band through the middle so that it can be used in a seated position.

Extend arms in front of the body and hold the band with a neutral grip (Figure 3.30).

Action: Retract the scapulae; lead with the elbows and pull the band back toward the sides of the torso in line with the sternum (Figure 3.31). Hold for several seconds, release, and slowly return to the starting position.

Common errors:

Error: Raising the shoulders

Correction: Keep the shoulders down and shoulder blades in neutral position.

Error: Flexing at the wrist

Correction: Pull in a straight line with straight wrists through the entire range of motion.

Variations:

• Single arm

• Low row (the ending point is at belly button-level and the arms can be supinated)

• Seated on bench

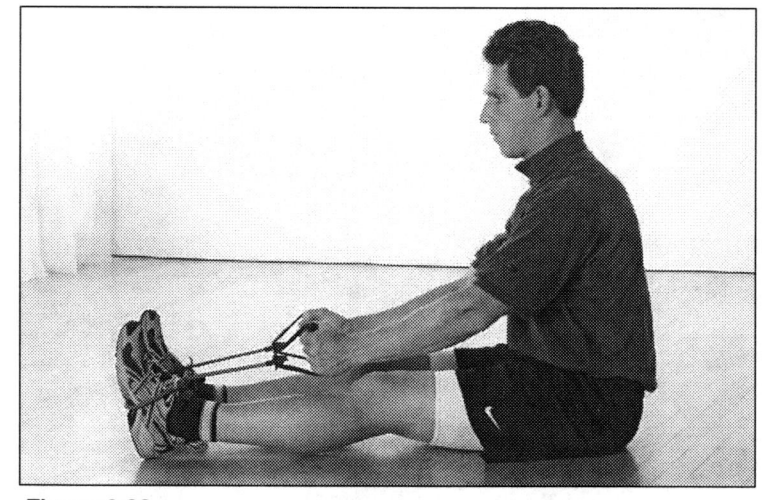

Figure 3.30
Seated row; starting position

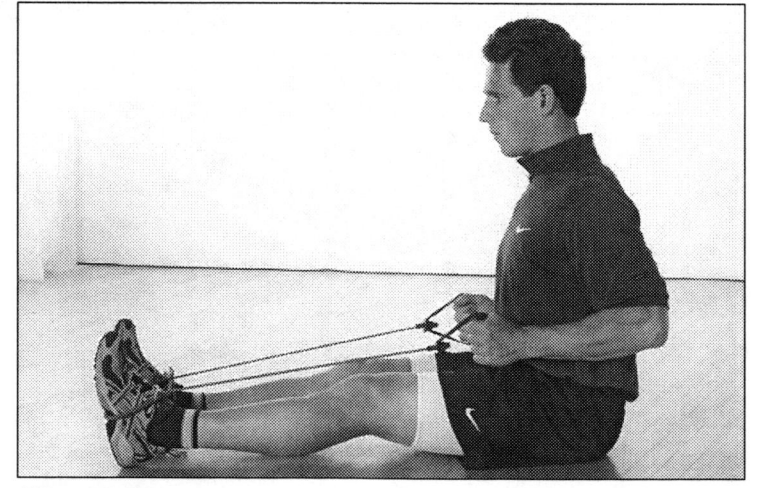

Figure 3.31
Seated row; action

Shoulders

Muscles involved:
Anterior, posterior,
and middle deltoid

Strength-training techniques for the shoulder:

1. Avoid exercises that exceed 90 degrees of shoulder flexion or extension. Front and side lateral raises should start with the arms slightly in front of the body and lift to no more than 90 degrees of shoulder abduction or flexion. This starting position and movement action help to protect the shoulder joint.

2. To protect the shoulder joint, overhead shoulder presses should be done in front of the body rather than behind the neck.

3. When pressing over the head, keep the spine neutral with the abdominals contracted to support the torso.

4. Rows performed with the elbows closer to the body target the latissimus dorsi, rhomboids, and biceps. Rows performed with the shoulders abducted target the rhomboids, posterior deltoid, and middle trapezius.

Table 3.3
Exercises for the Shoulder

Position	Resistance	Exercises
Standing	Weights	Front deltoid raise Lateral deltoid raise Overhead press Posterior shoulder extension
Standing	Elastic	Front deltoid raise Lateral deltoid raise Overhead press Posterior shoulder extension
Seated	Weights	Front deltoid raise Lateral deltoid raise Overhead press Posterior shoulder extension
All-fours	Weights	Single-arm posterior shoulder extension

Front Deltoid Raise

Targeted muscle: Anterior deltoid

Starting position: Arms start in front of the body with the palms facing the thighs. Engage the abdominals, bend the knees slightly, and position the feet about shoulder-width apart (Figure 3.32).

Action: With the elbows extended, flex at the shoulders to raise the arms to 90 degrees (i.e., to shoulder height) (Figure 3.33). Pause, then slowly return to the starting position.

Common error:

Error: Raising the arms too high

Correction: Stop the hands when they reach shoulder height, before they get to eye level.

Variation:

• Single arm (Figure 3.34)

Equipment variations:

• Elastic resistance anchored at the feet

• Seated on a bench or ball

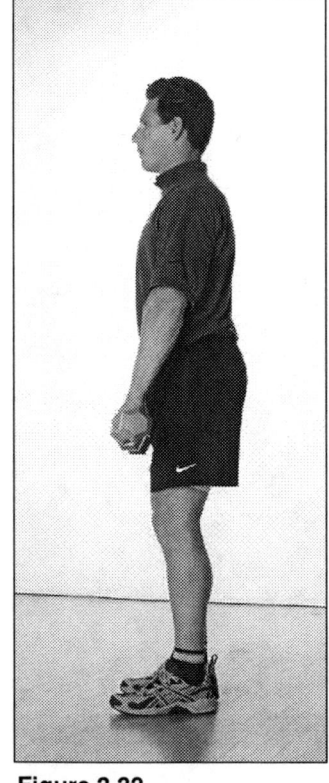

Figure 3.32
Front deltoid raise;
starting position

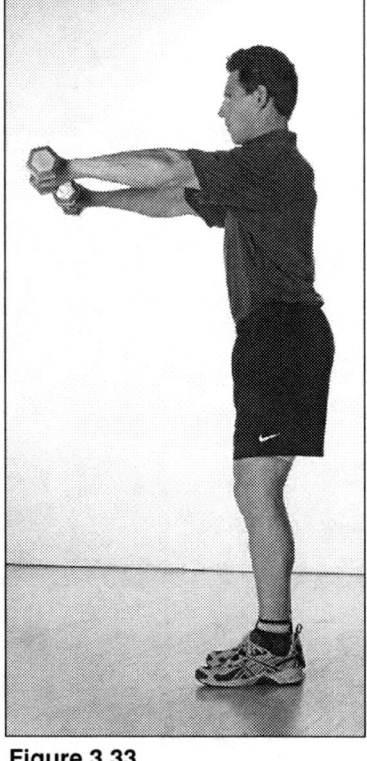

Figure 3.33
Front deltoid raise;
action

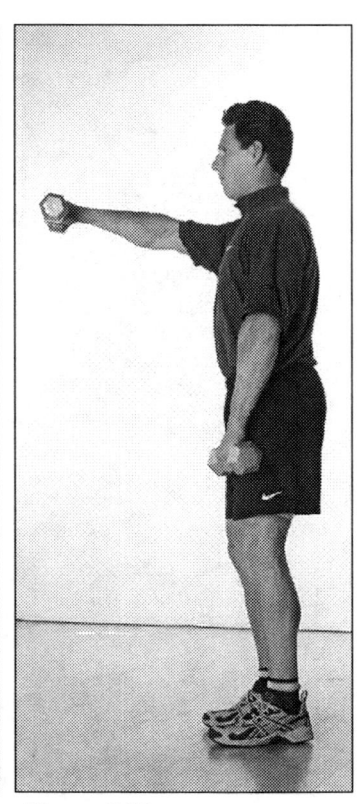

Figure 3.34
Front deltoid raise variation;
single-arm

Lateral Deltoid Raise

Targeted muscles: Anterior, middle, and posterior deltoid

Starting position: Arms start slightly anterior to the body, palms facing the thighs. This starting position helps protect the shoulder joint. Engage the abdominals, bend the knees slightly, and position the feet about shoulder-width apart (Figure 3.35).

Action: Keep elbows slightly flexed and abduct at the shoulders to raise the arms 90 degrees (i.e., to shoulder height) (Figure 3.36). Pause, then slowly return to the starting position.

Common error:

Error: Raising the arms too high

Correction: Stop the elbows when they reach shoulder height.

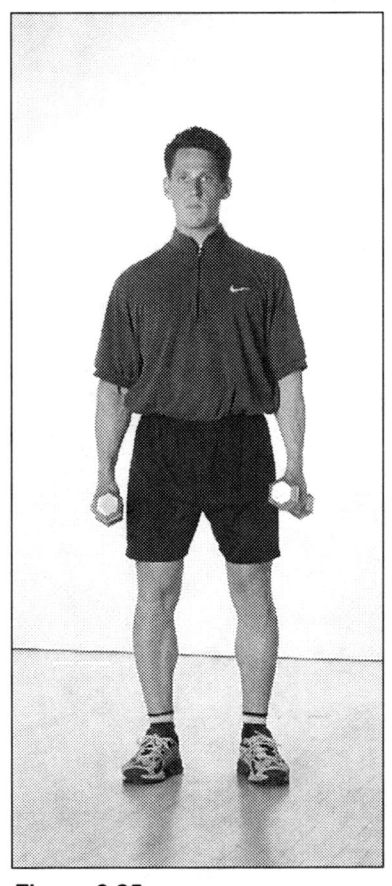

Figure 3.35
Lateral deltoid raise;
starting position

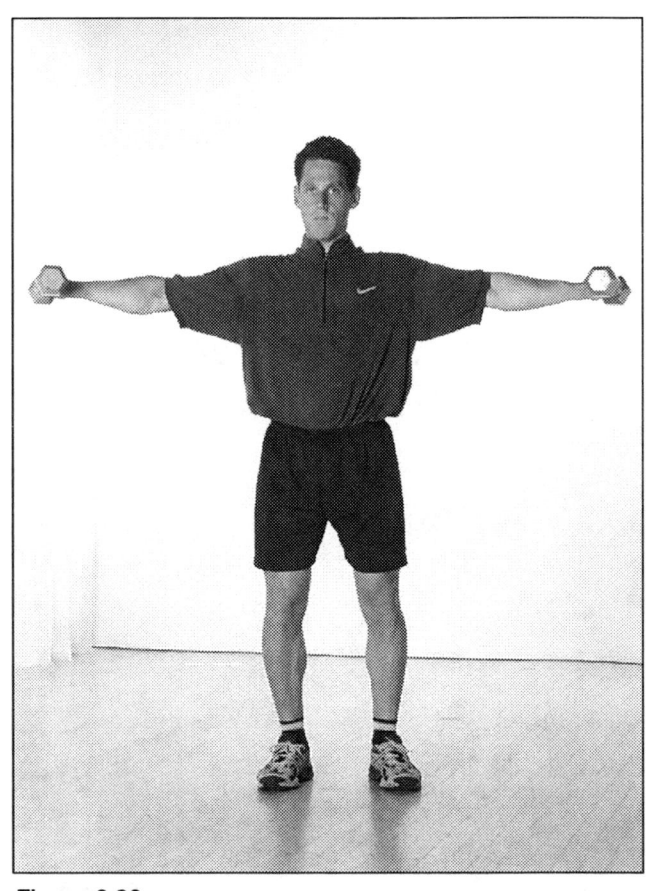

Figure 3.36
Lateral deltoid raise; action

Variations:

- Single arm
- Flex the elbows to reduce the intensity
  (Figure 3.37)

Equipment variations:

- Elastic resistance anchored under feet
- Seated on a bench or ball

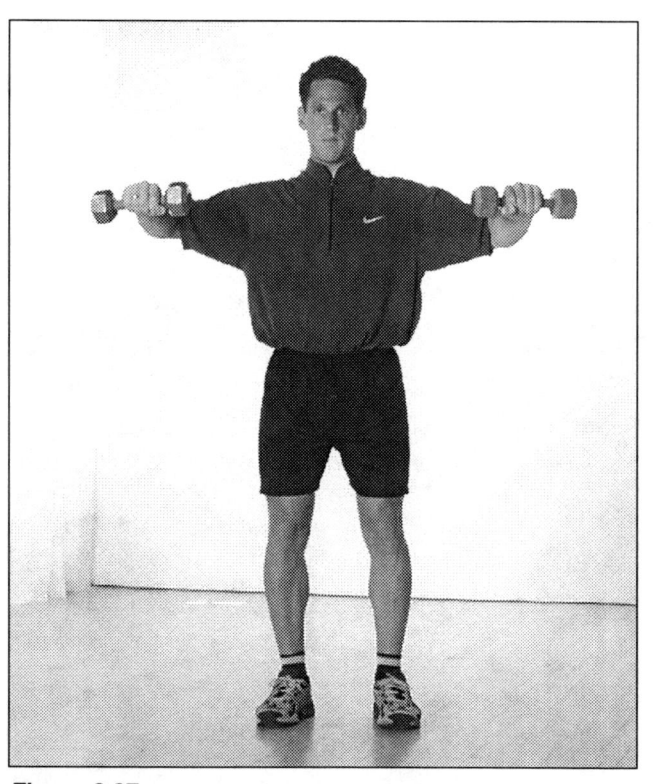

Figure 3.37
Lateral deltoid raise variation; flex
the elbows to reduce intensity

Overhead Press

Targeted muscles: Middle deltoid, triceps

Starting position: Hands start slightly above shoulder height, elbows flexed. Engage the abdominals, bend the knees slightly, and position the feet about shoulder-width apart (Figure 3.38).

Action: Abduct at the shoulders and press the hands over the head until elbows are extended but not locked (Figure 3.39). Pause, then slowly return to the starting position.

Common errors:

Error: Hands drifting behind the neck; elbows drifting behind the shoulders

Correction: Keep arms slightly in front of the ears to prevent hyperextension of the spine.

Error: Spine moving into hyperextension as weights are lifted above the head

Correction: Keep the abdominals engaged to stabilize neutral spine.

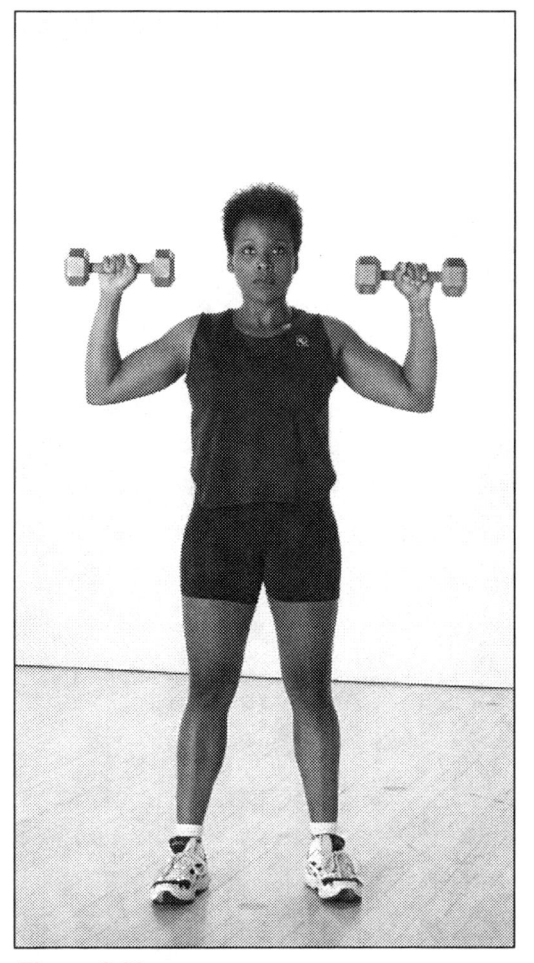

Figure 3.38
Overhead press; starting position

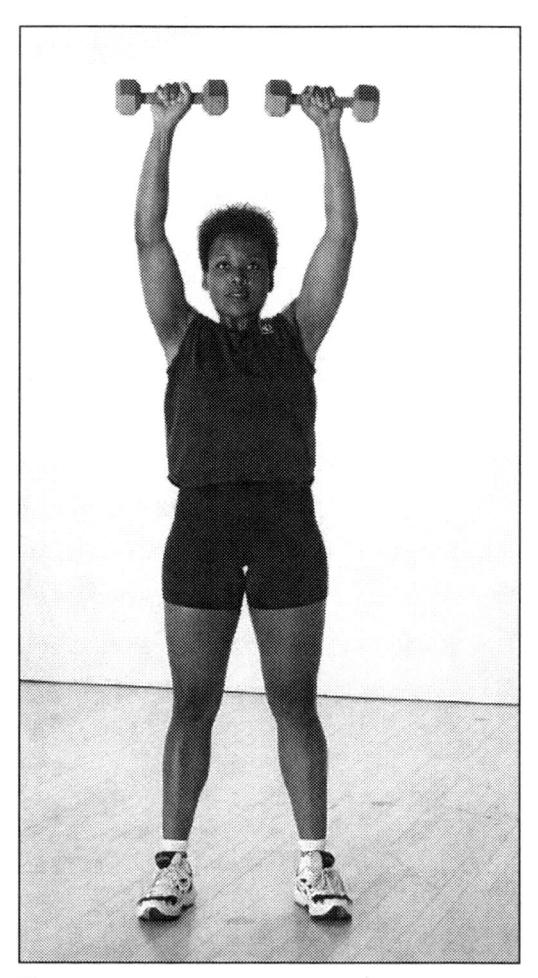

Figure 3.39
Overhead press; action

Variations:

• Arnold press, in which the hands pronate during the lifting phase and supinate during the lowering phase (Figure 3.40)

• Single arm

Equipment variations:

• Elastic resistance secured at the feet

• Seated on a bench or ball

• Elastic resistance with a single arm, with the band secured under the same foot

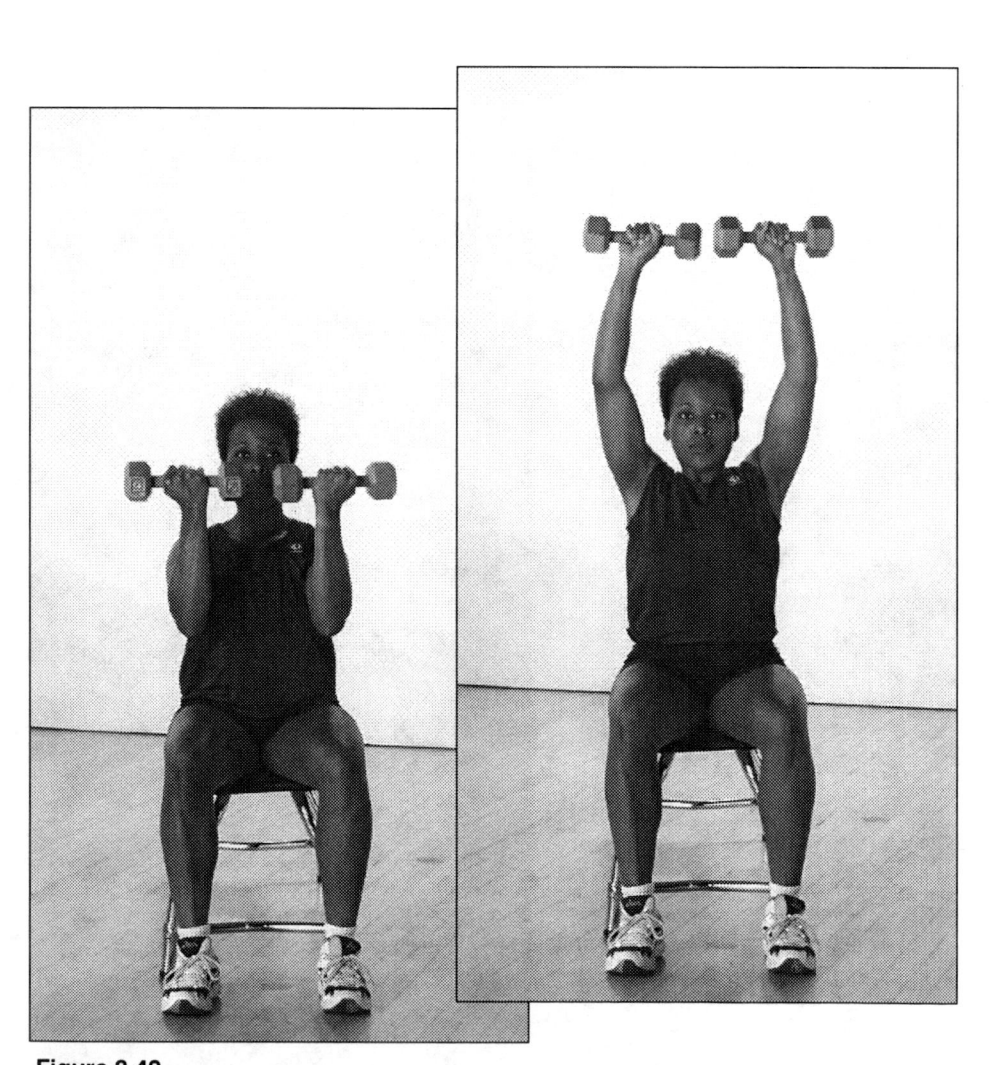

Figure 3.40
Overhead press variation; Arnold press

Posterior Shoulder Extension

Targeted muscle: Posterior deltoid

Starting position: Start in lunge position, lean the torso forward to 45 degrees, and provide additional support for the back with the non-working hand on the forward leg, with the arm rotated inward so the fingers are toward the inner thigh. Extend the working arm toward the floor with the palm facing the non-working hand. Engage the abdominals to help maintain neutral spine (Figure 3.41).

Action: Retract the scapula and, keeping the elbow extended, abduct the arm 90 degrees (i.e., to shoulder height) (Figure 3.42). Pause, then slowly lower weight to the starting position.

Common errors:

Error: Not supporting the lower back

Correction: Place the non-working hand firmly on the mid-thigh.

Error: Twisting the torso, raising the shoulder

Correction: Keep the shoulders stationary and even.

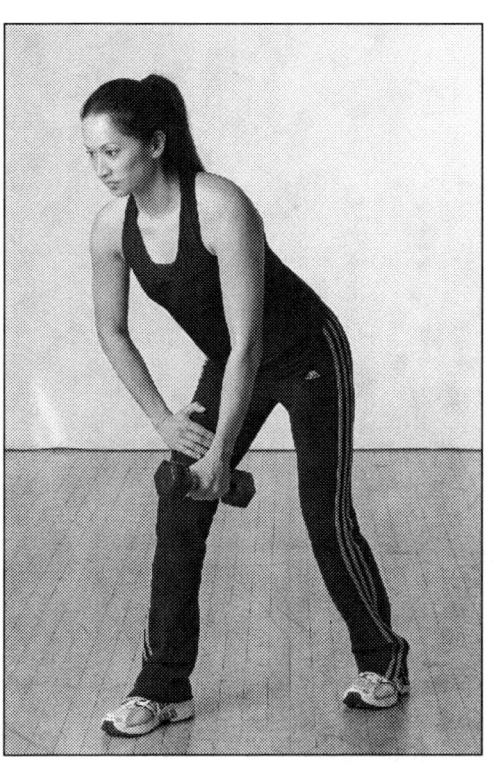

Figure 3.41
Posterior shoulder extension; starting position

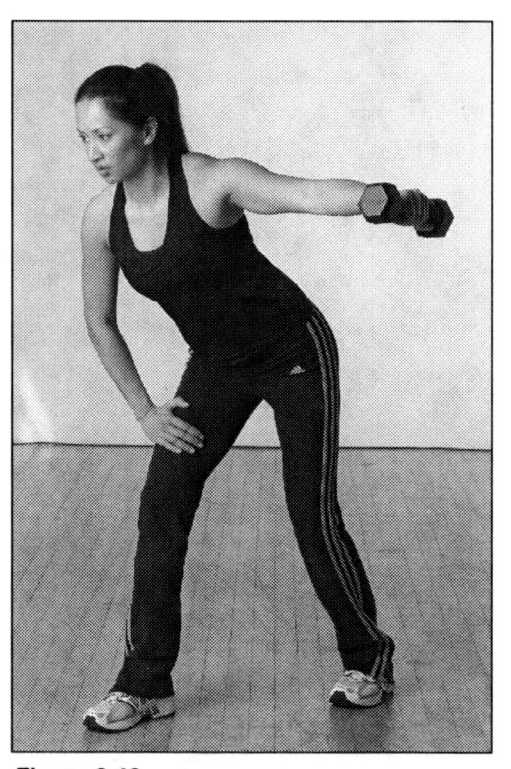

Figure 3.42
Posterior shoulder extension; action

Variation:

• On hands and knees, single-arm lifts with weight (Figure 3.43)

Equipment variations:

• Elastic resistance in staggered stance with band anchored at front foot

• Elastic resistance from seated position (on a bench or ball) with band anchored at feet

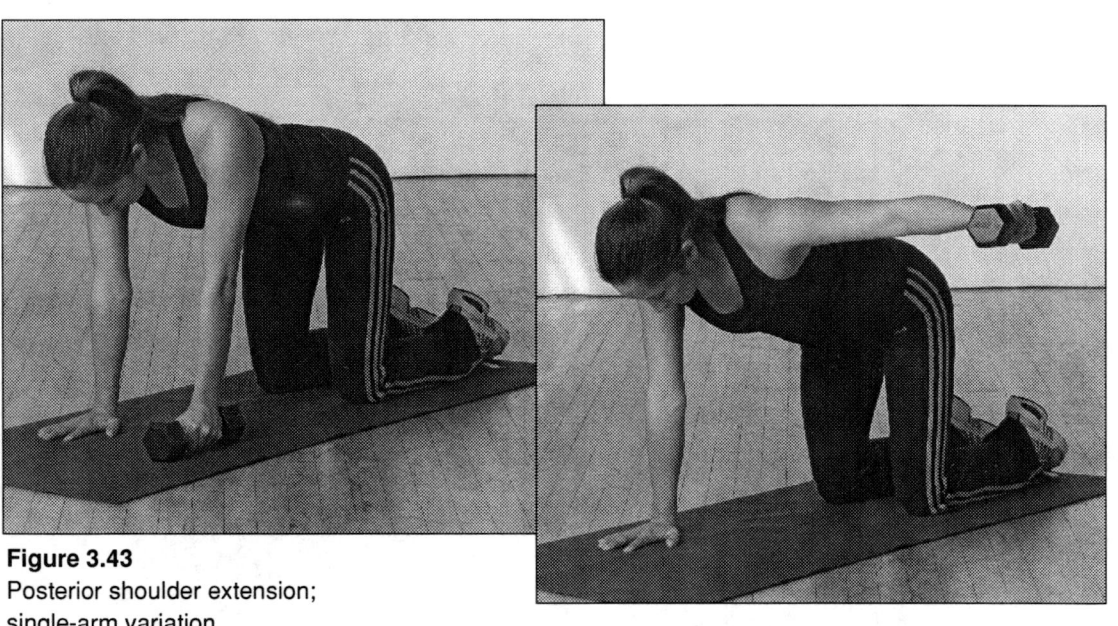

Figure 3.43
Posterior shoulder extension;
single-arm variation

Rotator Cuff

Muscles involved: Infraspinatus, subscapularis, supraspinatus, teres minor

Strength-training technique for the rotator cuff:

Teach participants how to stabilize, or set, the upper body to eliminate extra movement in the shoulders, back, and spine. Have them lightly retract their shoulder blades and maintain a neutral spine throughout these exercises.

External Shoulder Rotation

Targeted muscles: Infraspinatus, teres minor

Starting position: Flex both elbows 90 degrees, holding the upper arms next to the torso (Figure 3.44).

Action: Externally rotate both arms through full range of motion (Figure 3.45). Pause, then slowly return to the starting position.

Table 3.4
Exercises for the Rotator Cuff

Position	Resistance	Exercises
Standing	Elastic	External shoulder extension
Seated	Elastic	External shoulder extension
		Internal shoulder extension
Side-lying	Weights	External shoulder extension

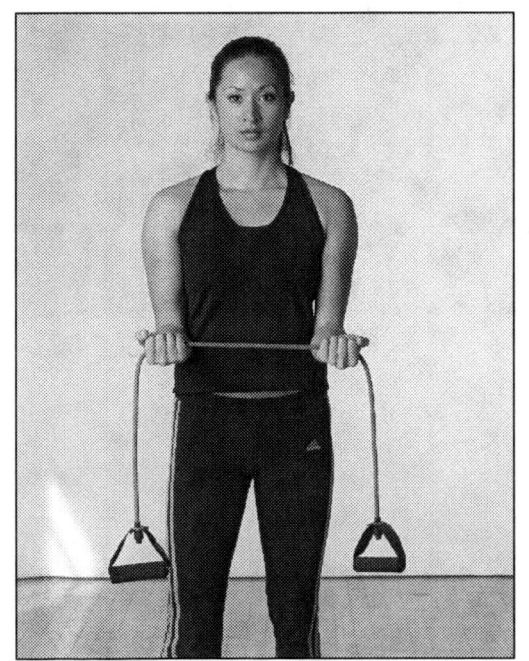

Figure 3.44
External shoulder rotation; starting position

Figure 3.45
External shoulder rotation; action

Common errors:

Error: Rotating the torso

Correction: Keep the body stationary.

Error: Upper arm drifting away from body

Correction: Hold a towel between the elbow and the ribs.

Variation:

• Side-lying with weights (Figure 3.46)

Equipment variations:

• Standing in a staggered lunge position with the non-moving arm providing additional support for the lower back

• Seated with elastic resistance anchored to opposite foot

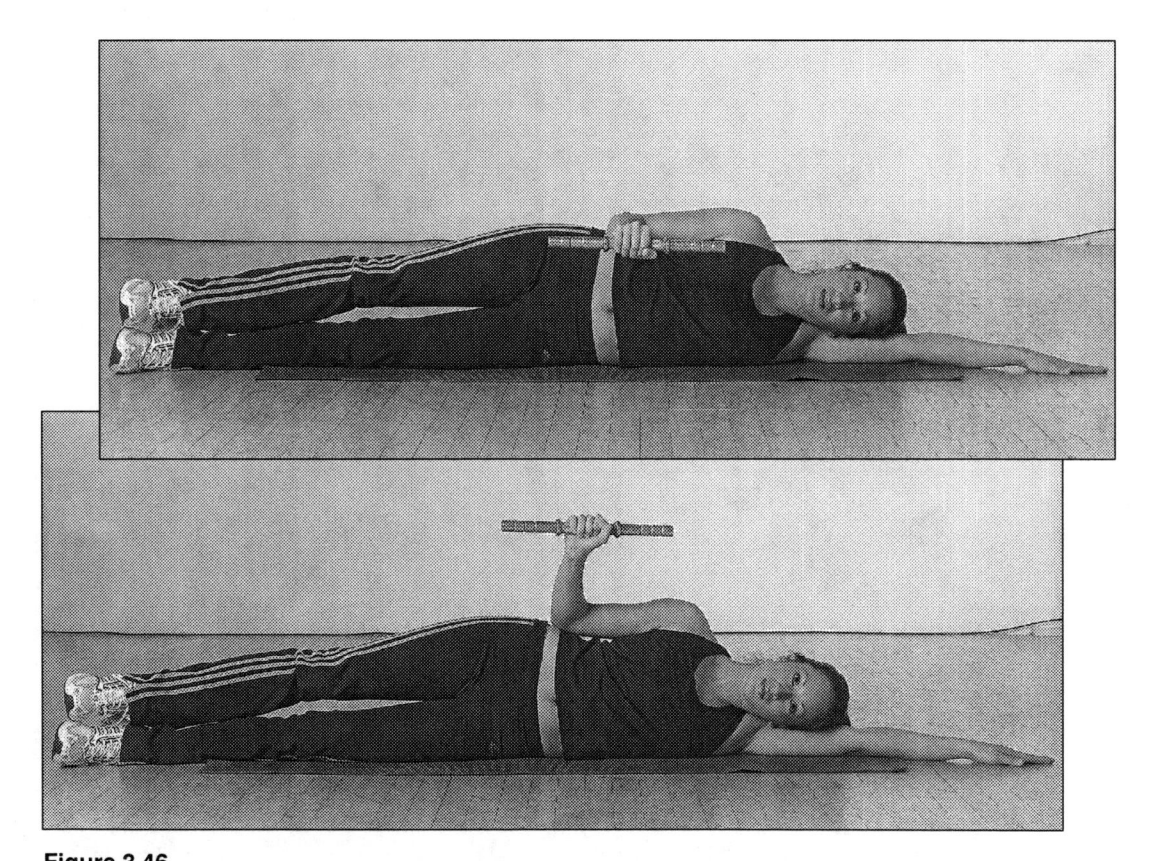

Figure 3.46
External shoulder rotation; side-lying variation

Internal Shoulder Rotation

Targeted muscle: Subscapularis

Starting position: Sit with one leg extended and the elastic resistance wrapped around the extended foot. If the right leg is extended, the left hand acts to anchor the elastic resistance and the right arm is bent 90 degrees with the upper arm next to the torso and slightly in front of the body (Figure 3.47).

Action: Internally rotate the right hand toward the body (Figure 3.48). Pause, then slowly return to the starting position. Repeat with the other arm.

Common errors:

Error: Rotating the torso

Correction: Keep the body stationary.

Error: Upper arm drifting away from body

Correction: Hold a towel between the elbow and the ribs.

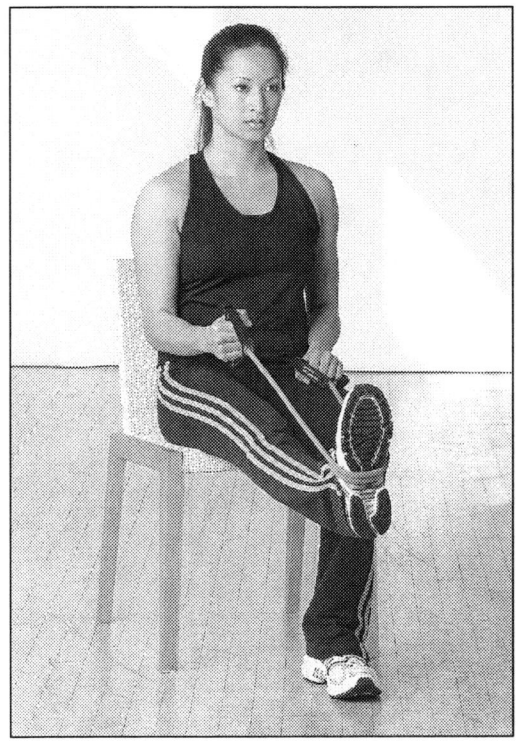

Figure 3.47
Internal shoulder rotation;
starting position

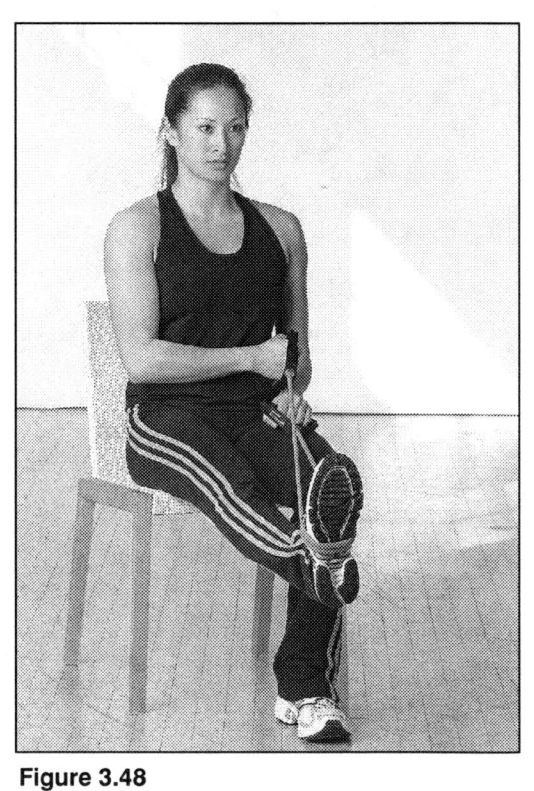

Figure 3.48
Internal shoulder rotation;
action

Triceps

Muscle involved: Triceps
Strength-training techniques
for the triceps:

1. Deep elbow flexion may cause excessive stress on the elbow joint during triceps exercises.

Table 3.5
Exercises for the Triceps

Position	Resistance	Exercises
Standing	Weights	Overhead triceps press
		Triceps kick-back
Standing	Elastic	Overhead triceps press
		Triceps kick-back
Seated	Weights	Overhead triceps press
Seated	Bodyweight	Bench dips

2. When pressing over the head, engage the abdominals to help maintain neutral spine.

Bench Dip

Targeted muscle: Triceps

Starting position: Sit on a bench and grip the front edge with hands shoulder-width apart. Extend the legs straight in front of the body with the heels on the floor. Move forward until the hips are off the bench (Figure 3.49).

Action: Slowly lower the hips toward the floor, then press up to full arm extension without locking the elbows (Figure 3.50).

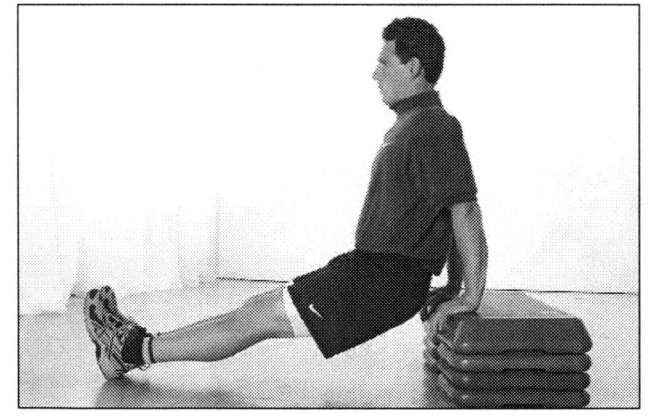

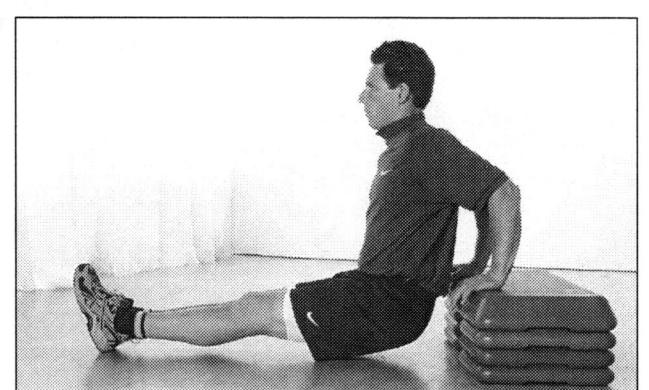

Figure 3.49
Bench dip; starting position

Figure 3.50
Bench dip; action

45

Common errors:

Error: Descending too deeply

Correction: Descend only until the upper arm is parallel to the floor; this protects the anterior shoulder capsule.

Error: Lowering too fast

Correction: Slowly count to four while lowering the body.

Error: Shoulders internally rotating and rounding forward during descent

Correction: Slightly retract the scapulae to keep the anterior shoulder girdle in good neutral alignment.

Error: Elbows flare outward

Correction: Keep elbows angled rearward.

Error: Hips move increasingly farther away from the edge of the bench

Correction: Position the legs so the hips can remain very close to the bench throughout the movement.

Variations:

• Begin with bent knees with the feet directly beneath the knees to reduce workload.

• Place a weight securely on the upper-thigh area to increase workload.

Equipment variation:

• Feet can be placed on a second bench (Figure 3.51). This increases intensity by increasing the effects of gravity and overall workload.

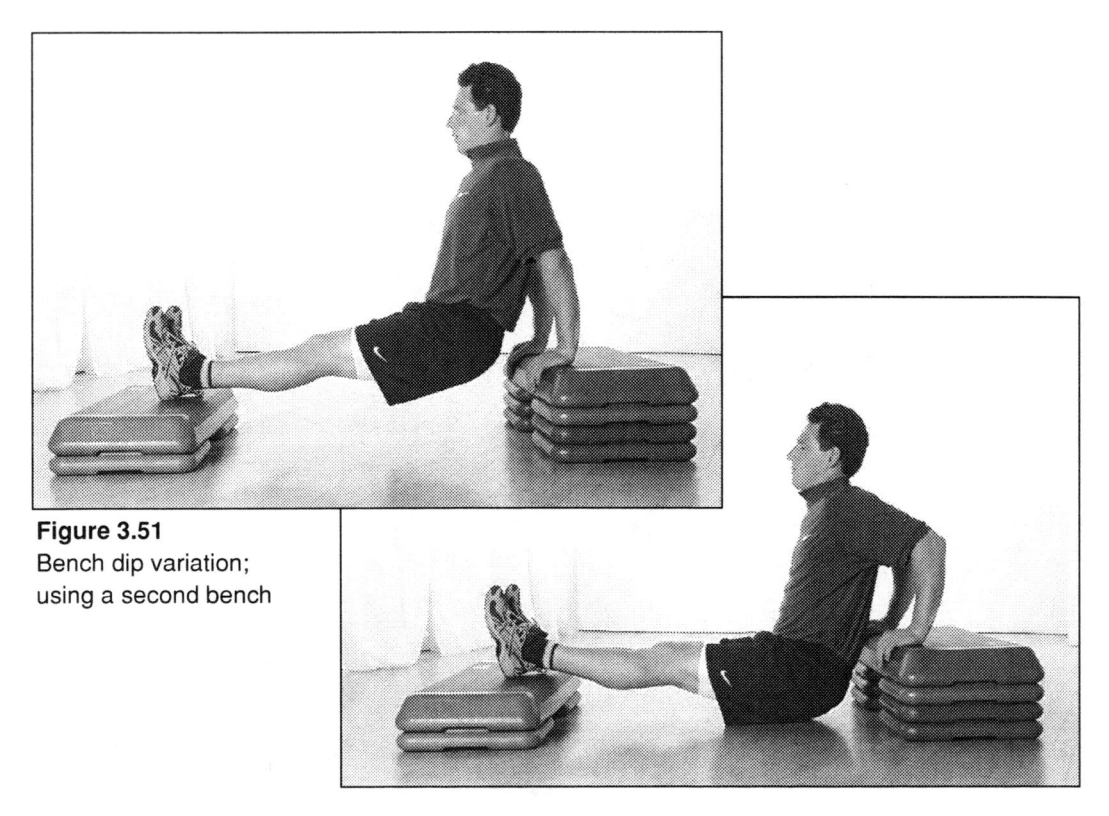

Figure 3.51
Bench dip variation;
using a second bench

Overhead Triceps Press

Targeted muscle: Triceps

Starting position: Stand erect with elbows aligned with the shoulders just above the ears. Hold a weight slightly above the scapula. Keep the upper arm stationary throughout the entire exercise (Figure 3.52).

Action: Extend the elbows and lift the weight above the head to the point just prior to locking the elbows (Figure 3.53). Pause, then slowly lower the weight until the forearms are parallel to the floor.

Common errors:

Error: Upper-arm movement

Correction: Keep the upper arm stationary as though it is part of the spine.

Error: Elbows flare outward

Correction: Keep elbows close to ears.

Error: Spine moving into hyperextension as weights are lifted above the head

Correction: Keep the abdominals engaged to stabilize neutral spine.

Variations:

• Single arm

• Staggered foot position

Equipment variations:

• Elastic resistance

• Seated on a bench or on the floor

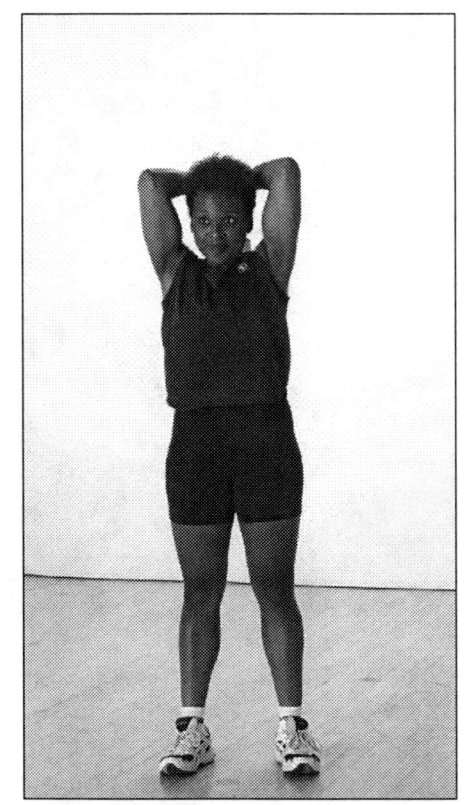

Figure 3.52
Overhead triceps press; starting position

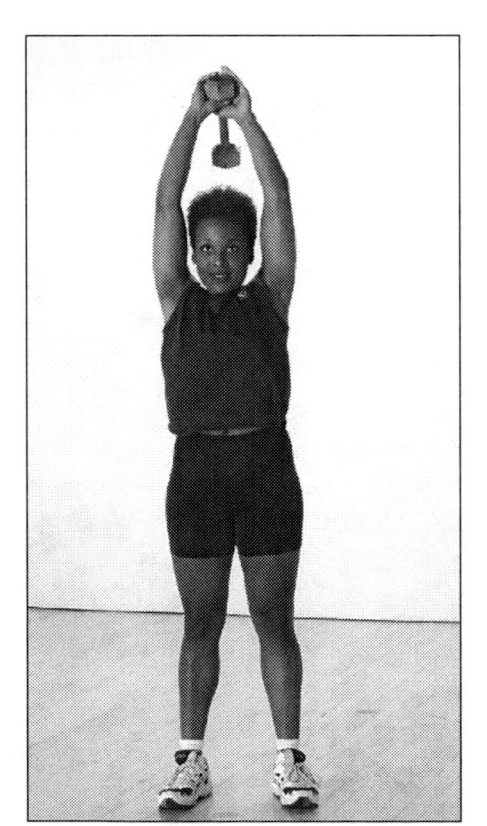

Figure 3.53
Overhead triceps press; action

Triceps Kick-back

Targeted muscle: Triceps

Starting position: Begin with feet in a staggered position. Provide additional support for the trunk by placing one hand on the thigh with a slightly bent elbow and the arm rotated inward so the fingers are toward the inner thigh. With the weight in the other hand, extend the shoulder rearward until the upper arm is parallel with the floor, the elbow is flexed, and the palm is facing the torso. Engage the abdominals (Figure 3.54).

Action: Contract the triceps until the elbow almost fully extends (Figure 3.55). Pause, then slowly return to the starting position.

Common errors:

Error: Moving the upper arm

Correction: Keep the upper arm stationary throughout the entire movement.

Error: Swinging the weight

Correction: Slowly lower the weight back to the starting position and pause when the hand returns to a position under the elbow.

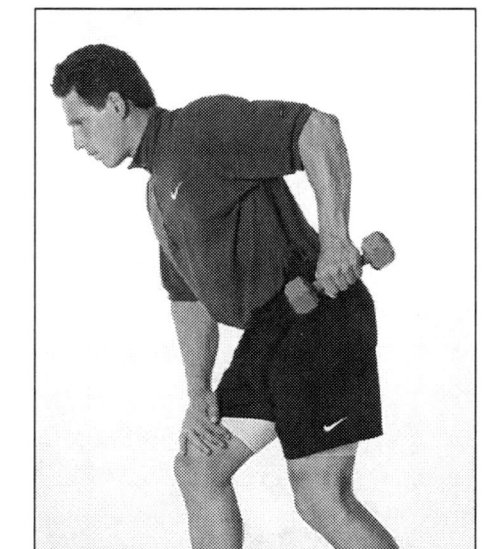

Figure 3.54
Triceps kick-back; starting position

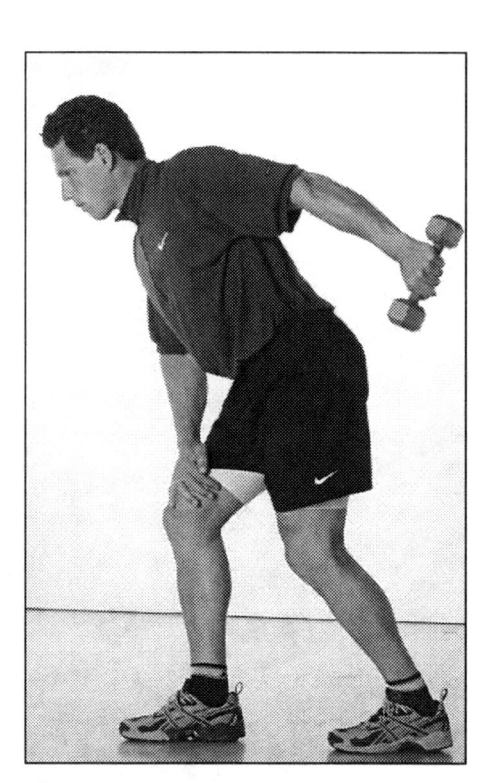

Figure 3.55
Triceps kick-back; action

Variations:

• Start with feet shoulder-width apart rather than staggered. Maintaining a neutral spine, flex forward at the hips 30 degrees and perform the exercise with both arms at the same time (Figure 3.56).

• Use a bench to support body weight on one knee and hand.

Equipment variation:

• Elastic resistance (Figure 3.57)

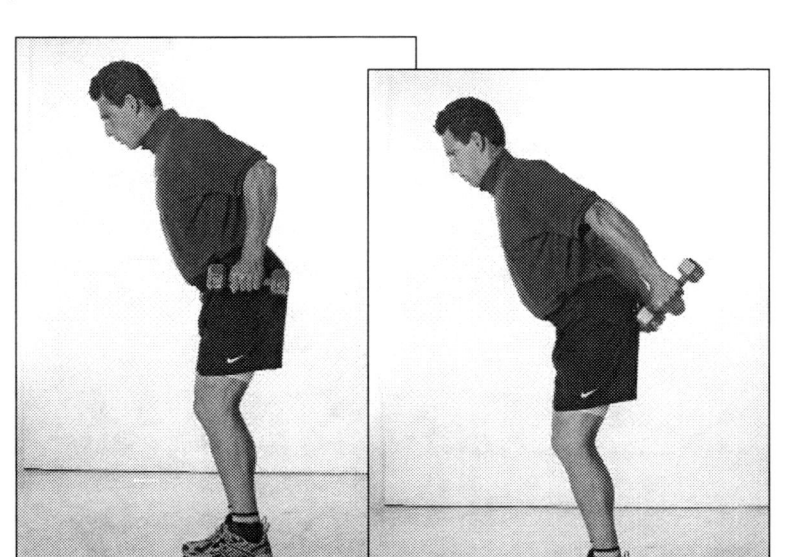

Figure 3.56
Triceps kick-back
variation

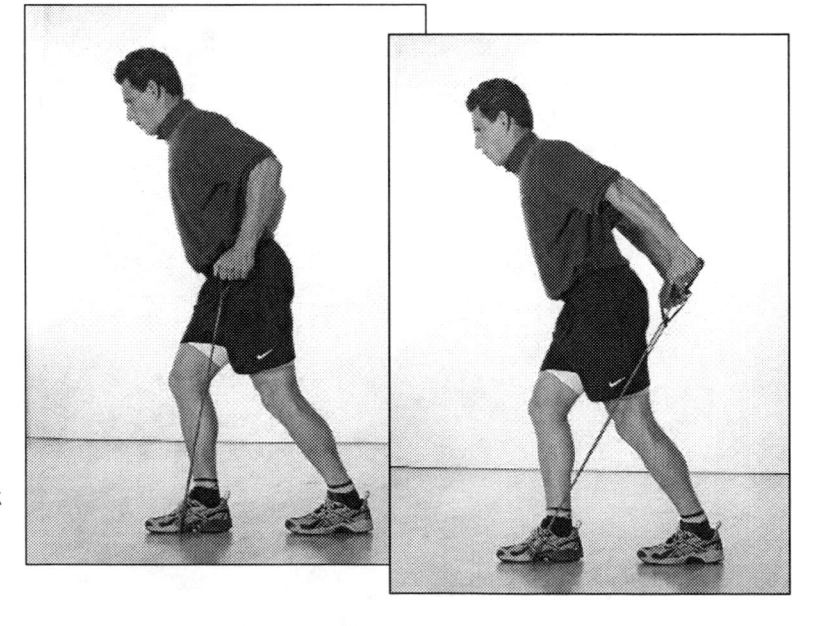

Figure 3.57
Triceps kick-back
variation; elastic
resistance

Biceps

Muscles involved:
Biceps, brachialis,
brachioradialis

Strength-training technique for the biceps:
Avoid overgripping weights or elastic resistance, which fatigues the forearms isometrically and can elevate blood pressure.

Biceps Curl

Targeted muscle: Biceps

Starting position: Stand erect with the knees slightly bent and engage the abdominals to help maintain neutral spine. Arms hang down along the sides of the body with the palms facing forward (Figure 3.58).

Action: Simultaneously curl both dumbbells up to shoulder height (Figure 3.59). Pause, then slowly lower arms to the starting position.

Common errors:

Error: Swinging arms or elbows

Correction: Stabilize the elbows directly under the shoulders and next to the torso throughout the movement.

Error: Overgripping the weight

Table 3.6
Exercises for the Biceps

Position	Resistance	Exercises
Standing	Weights	Biceps curl
Seated	Weights	Biceps curl

Correction: Gently grasp the weight so there is no chance of dropping it.

Variations:

• Seated on the end of a bench

• Single arm

• Begin with the palm facing the side of the body and supinate the lower arm during the lift.

• Begin with the palm facing the side of the body and maintain that position throughout the exercise (hammer curl).

• Pronate the wrist (i.e., the palm is facing posteriorly) and maintain that position throughout the exercise (reverse curl).

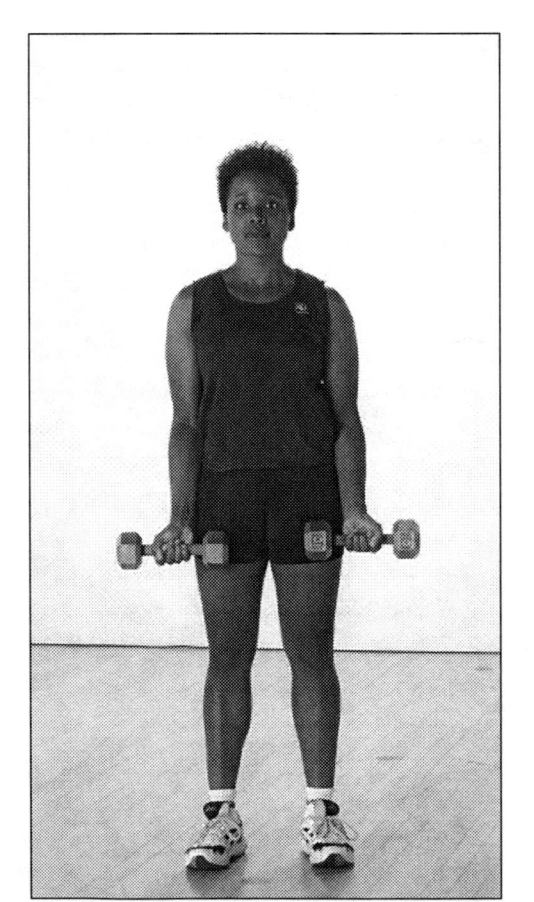

Figure 3.58
Biceps curl; starting position

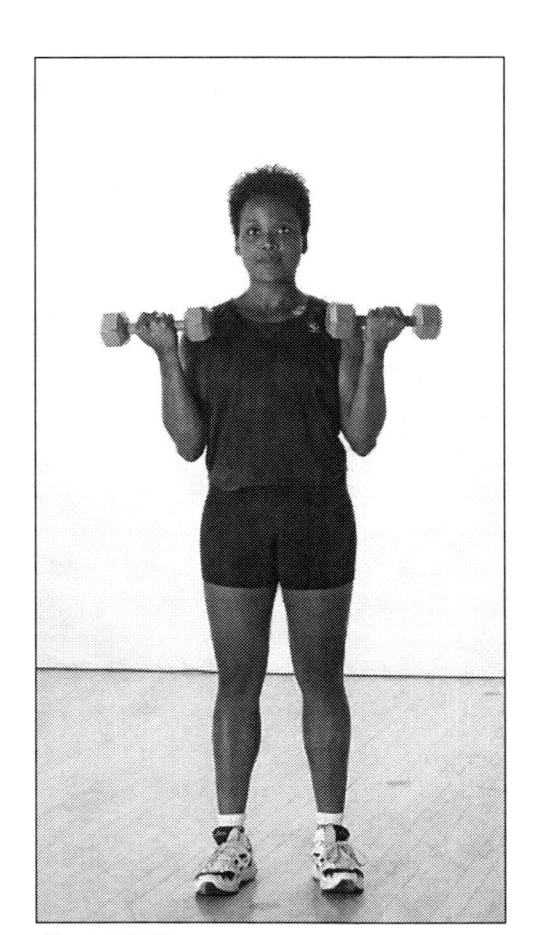

Figure 3.59
Biceps curl; action

Torso

Muscles involved: Rectus abdominis, internal obliques, external obliques, erector spinae

Strength-training techniques for the torso:

1. Keep the knees slightly bent to maintain neutral spinal alignment. This allows the pelvis to have greater mobility to attain a supportive position.

2. To work the abdominals safely and effectively, participants should maintain a neutral pelvis while they flex the thoracic spine (i.e., the mid-back area), bringing the bottom ribs toward the hips.

3. Avoid flapping the arms, pulling on the neck, and other movements that decrease the workload on the abdominal muscles.

4. It is acceptable to perform a high number of repetitions of abdominal exercises in multiple sets on non-consecutive days.

5. Torso exercises can be modified by extending one or both arms to increase the lever length of the body.

6. Make sure stability balls are firmly in place to ensure safety and effectiveness.

Abdominal Curl

Targeted muscle: Rectus abdominis

Starting position: Lie supine with one knee bent with the foot flat on the floor and the other leg extended. Cross your arms over the chest or place them, unclasped, behind the head with the elbows out to the side. Maintain neutral alignment in the cervical spine (Figure 3.60).

Table 3.7
Exercises for the Torso

Position	Resistance	Exercise
All-fours (or on stability ball)	Bodyweight	Back extension
Supine	Bodyweight	Abdominal curl
		Single-leg reverse curl
Supine	Weights	Abdominal curl
Side-lying	Bodyweight	Side bridge

Action: Engage the abdominals and exhale while curling up. Initiate the movement by gently flexing the cervical spine by dropping the chin slightly. Next, activate the abdominals by raising the shoulders and upper back off the floor toward the pelvis. Contract at the top of the movement (Figure 3.61). Pause, then slowly return to the starting position.

Common errors:

Error: Forward neck position

Correction: Imagine an orange tucked between the chin and neck and maintain this position throughout the exercise.

Error: Moving the elbows forward while curling up

Correction: Keep elbows out of vision and remain open through the chest and shoulders.

Error: Holding the breath

Correction: Emphasize exhaling during the exertion phase.

Variation:

• Change arm position and lever length to increase or decrease intensity

Equipment variations:

• Dumbbells or weight plate held on the chest

• Decline with bench (advanced)

• Feet up on a bench

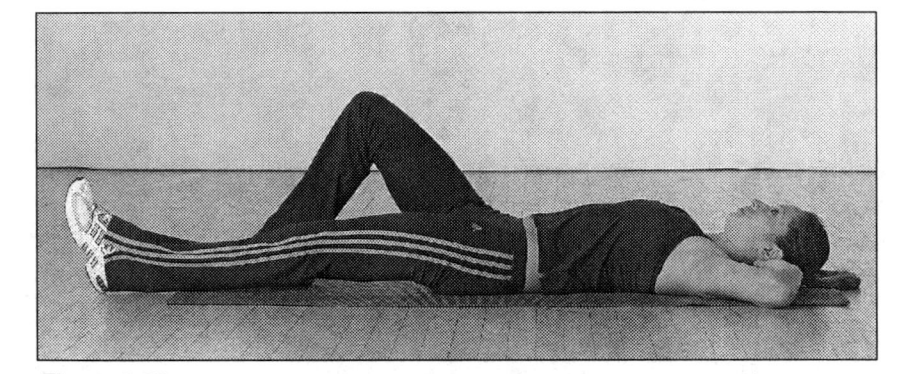

Figure 3.60
Abdominal curl;
starting position

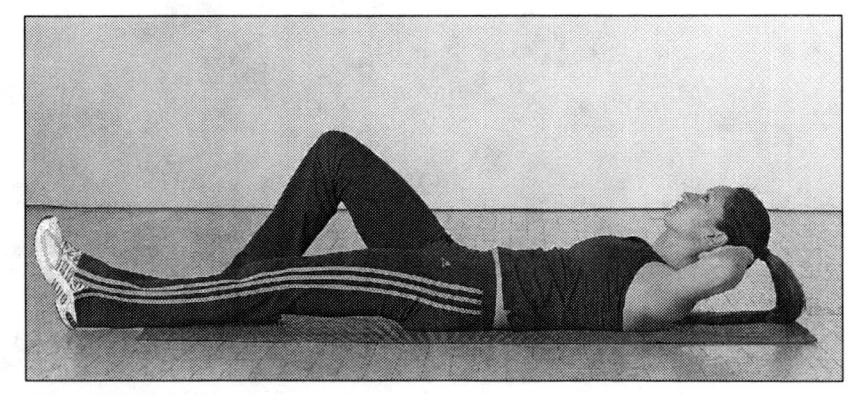

Figure 3.61
Abdominal curl; action

Side Bridge

Targeted muscle: External and internal obliques

Exercise position/action: Lie on one side with knees bent 90 degrees. Support the upper body by keeping the elbow directly beneath the shoulder. Being careful not to let the top hip rotate forward, engage the abdominals and use the torso to lift the hips (Figure 3.62). Hold this position for 10 to 15 seconds, maintaining a neutral neck and spine position.

Common errors:

Error: Dropping the hips

Correction: Slightly contract the gluteals and the abdominals to keep the body in good alignment.

Error: Twisting or tilting the head

Correction: Keep the head and neck aligned with the spine.

Variation:

• Extend the legs to increase the intensity (Figure 3.63).

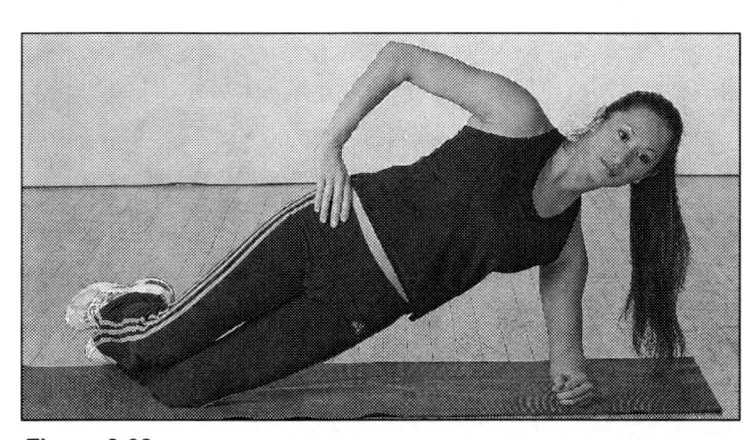

Figure 3.62
Side bridge; exercise position/action

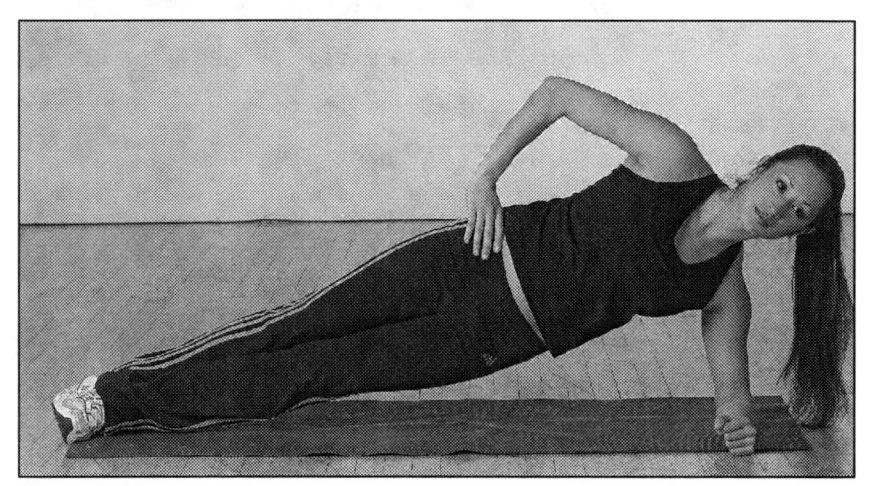

Figure 3.63
Side bridge variation; Extend the legs to increase intensity.

Single-leg Reverse Curl

Targeted muscle: Rectus abdominis

Starting position: Lie supine with one knee flexed and foot flat on the floor and the other hip flexed 90 degrees or more. Extend arms flat along body and maintain neutral alignment in the cervical spine (Figure 3.64).

Action: Lift the working knee and leg in an upward diagonal direction over the belly button (Figure 3.65). Pause, then slowly lower the leg to the starting position. Repeat with the other leg.

Common errors:

Error: Using hands or arms as leverage

Correction: Relax the arms, cross the arms over the chest, or turn the palms up.

Error: Holding the breath

Correction: Emphasize exhaling during the exertion phase.

Variation:

• Leg position: changing the angle of the hips or knees

Equipment variation:

• Incline with bench (advanced)

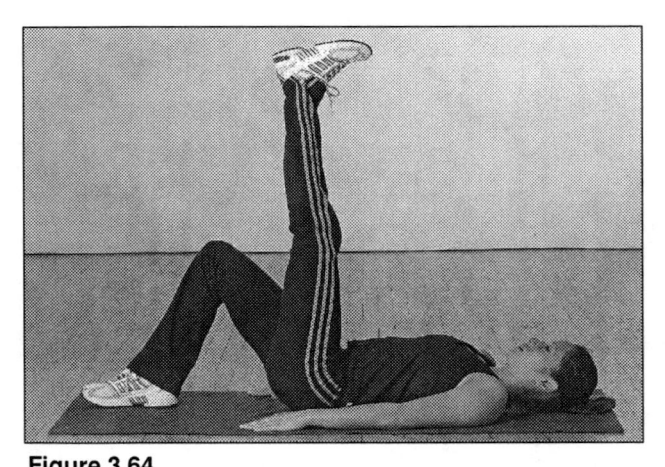

Figure 3.64
Single-leg reverse curl; starting position

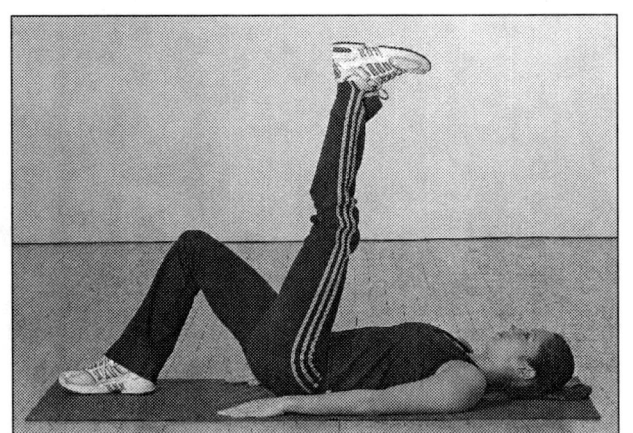

Figure 3.65
Single-leg reverse curl; action

Prone Back Extension

Targeted muscle: Erector spinae

Starting position: Begin in an all-fours position with the abdominal muscles engaged to stabilize the spine and pelvis and the neck in alignment with the spine (Figure 3.66).

Action: Lift the left arm and the right leg simultaneously (Figure 3.67). Pause, then slowly return to the starting position. Repeat on the opposite side.

Common errors:

Error: Holding the breath

Correction: Emphasize exhaling during the lifting phase of the exercise.

Error: Excessive extension of the lumbar and cervical spine

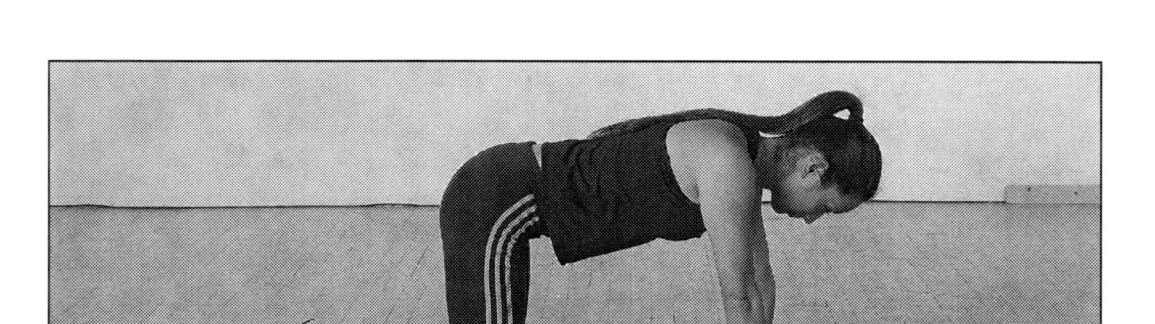

Figure 3.66
Prone back extension; starting position

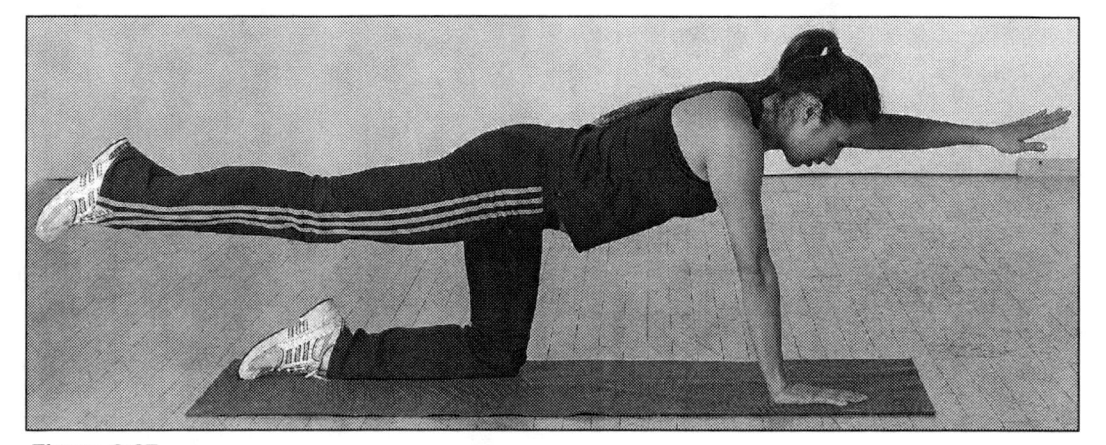

Figure 3.67
Prone back extension; action

Correction: Control the lifting phase and limit the range of motion of the neck and lower back, keeping the neck in alignment with the spine.

Error: Elevating the scapulae while extending the spine

Correction: Maintain neutral scapular position by gently sliding the scapulae downward while extending the spine.

Variations:

• Only upper body

• Change arm position and lever length to increase or decrease intensity

Equipment variations:

• Stability ball (Figure 3.68)

• Prone on bench

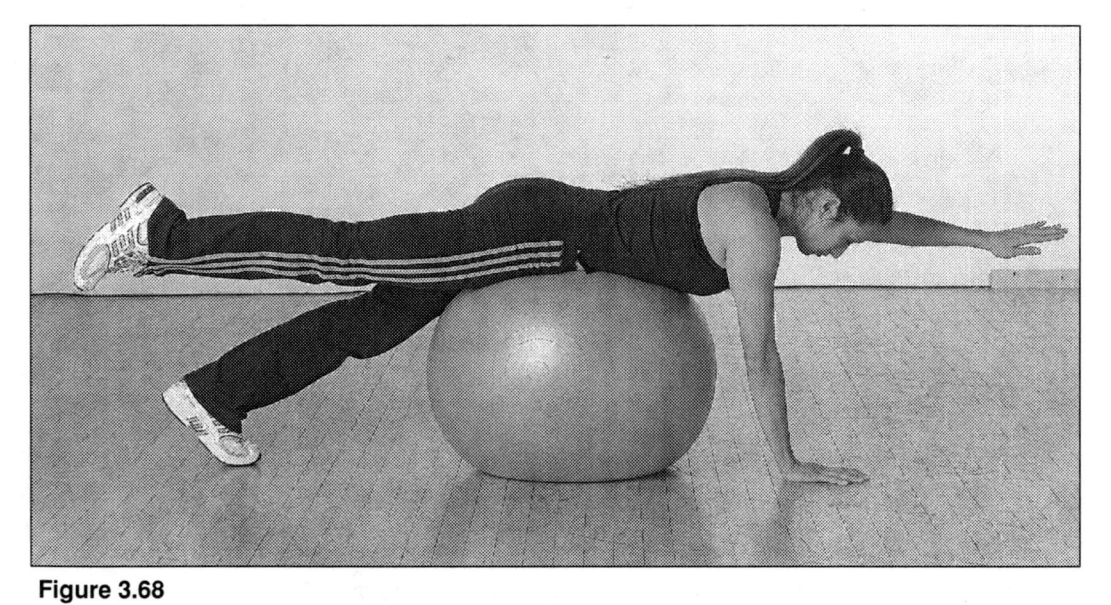

Figure 3.68
Prone back extension; variation using stability ball

Upper Legs and Hips

Muscles involved: Quadriceps, hamstrings, hip abductors, hip adductors, gluteals, hip flexors

Strength-training techniques for the upper legs and hips:

1. When using elastic resistance, placing the band above the knee creates less stress than placing the band below the knee.

2. During standing exercises, always keep the knees from gliding past the position directly over the ankles.

3. Stepping backward into a lunge places less stress on the knee than stepping forward into a lunge.

4. When strengthening the hips, engage the abdominals and keep the spine neutral.

Table 3.8

Exercises for the Upper Legs and Hips

Position	Resistance	Exercises
Standing	Weights + Elastic	Squat
Standing	Elastic	Straight-leg extension Outer thigh lift Inner thigh lift
Standing	Bodyweight	Squat Backward lunge Side lunge Front lunge Walking lunge Straight-leg extension Outer thigh lift
Seated	Elastic	Straight-leg extension
Seated	Bodyweight	Straight-leg extension
Prone	Bodyweight	Hip extension
Side-lying	Bodyweight	Outer thigh lift Inner thigh lift
Side-lying	Elastic	Outer thigh lift Inner thigh lift

Squat

Targeted muscles: Gluteals, hamstrings, quadriceps

Starting position: Stand erect with a neutral spine and feet shoulder-width apart (Figure 3.69).

Action: Slowly lower the body, with the hips moving back as if sitting in a chair. Maintain the weight directly over the heels or mid-foot. Lower to approximately 90 degrees of knee flexion (Figure 3.70). Pause, then slowly return to the starting position. If lumbar curvature cannot be maintained, lower less than 90 degrees.

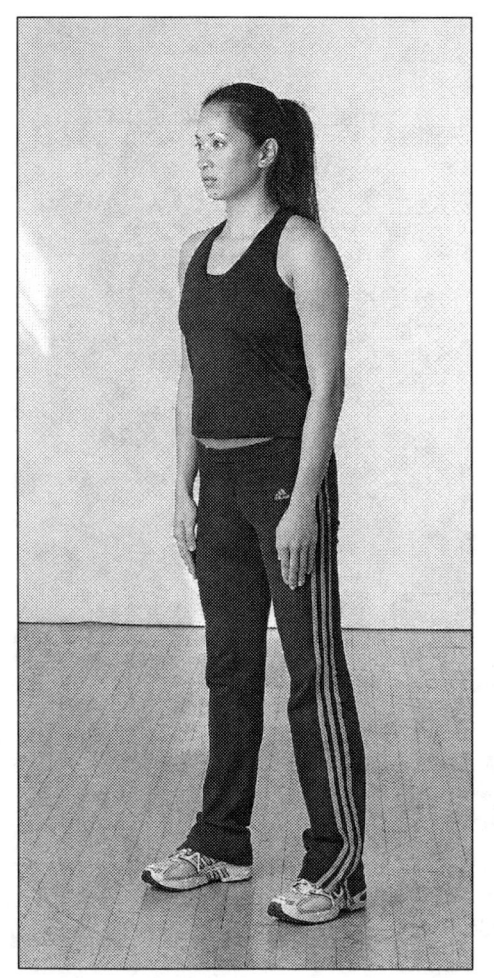

Figure 3.69
Squat; starting position

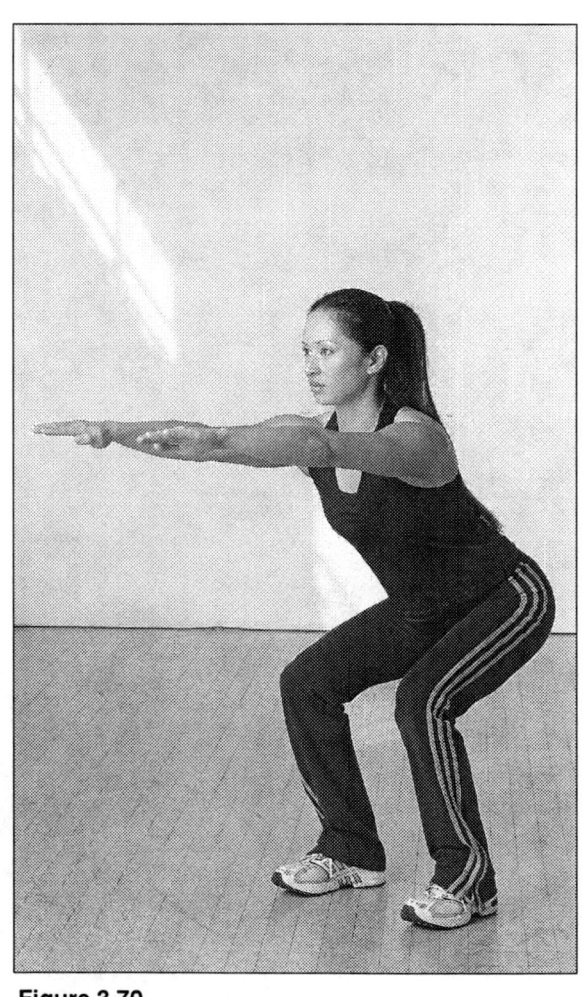

Figure 3.70
Squat; action

Common errors:

Error: Lowering beyond 90 degrees of flexion

Correction: Slowly lower the body and stop before the upper leg becomes parallel with the floor.

Error: Forward lean with heel lift

Correction: Keep the weight over the back portion of the foot rather than the toes; raise the arms to shoulder height to counterbalance.

Variation:

• One leg at a time

Equipment variation:

• Elastic resistance secured onto a straight bar (Figure 3.71)

• With small ball between the legs, to target the adductors (Figure 3.72)

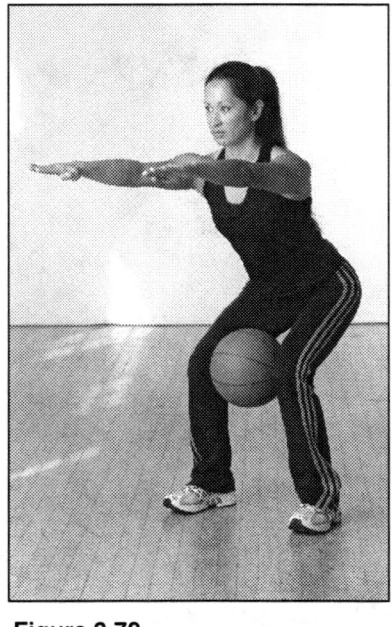

Figure 3.72
Squat variation; small ball between the legs to target the adductors

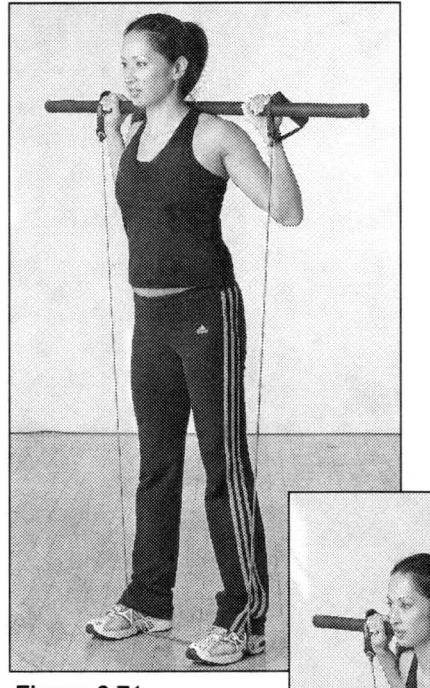

Figure 3.71
Squat variation; elastic resistance secured onto a straight bar

Backward Lunge

Targeted muscles: Gluteals, hamstrings, quadriceps

Starting position: Stand erect with a neutral spine and feet shoulder-width apart (Figure 3.73).

Action: Take a long step backward landing on the ball of the foot and bend the rear knee to a fencer's lunge position; lower to approximately 90 degrees of knee flexion (Figure 3.74). Pause, then return to the starting position. Maintain neutral spine throughout the movement. Repeat with the other leg.

Common errors:

Error: Dropping the head and shoulders forward
Correction: Keep the chest lifted over the top of the hips and look straight ahead with neck in neutral position.

Error: Lowering beyond 90 degrees of flexion
Correction: Slowly lower the body, and stop before the upper leg becomes parallel with the floor.

Error: Forward trunk lean with heel lift of lead leg
Correction: Keep the weight over the back portion of the foot rather than the toes; raise the arms to shoulder height to counterbalance.

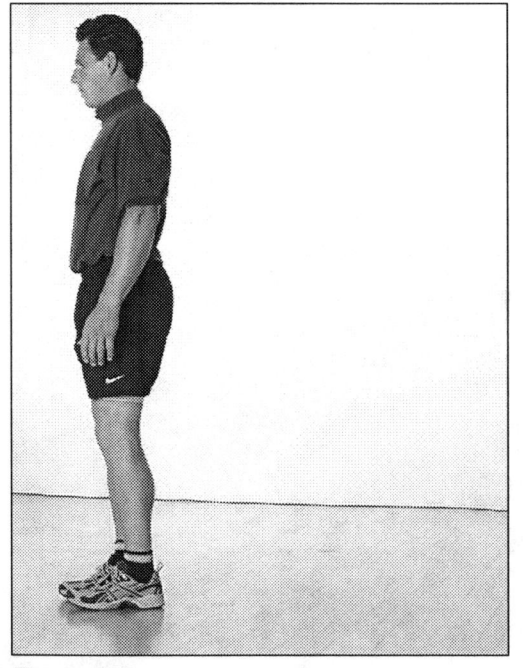

Figure 3.73
Backward lunge; starting position

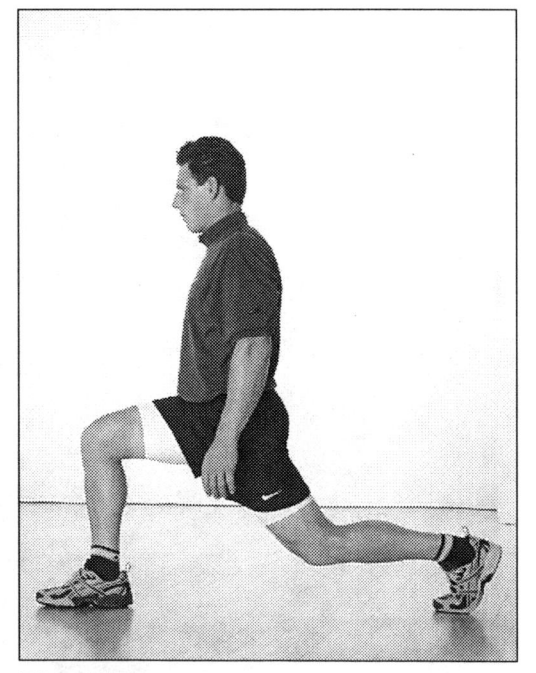

Figure 3.74
Backward lunge; action

Variations:

• Side lunge (Figure 3.75)

• Front lunge (Figure 3.76)

• Walking lunge

Equipment variations:

• Light hand or wrist weights

• Weighted vest

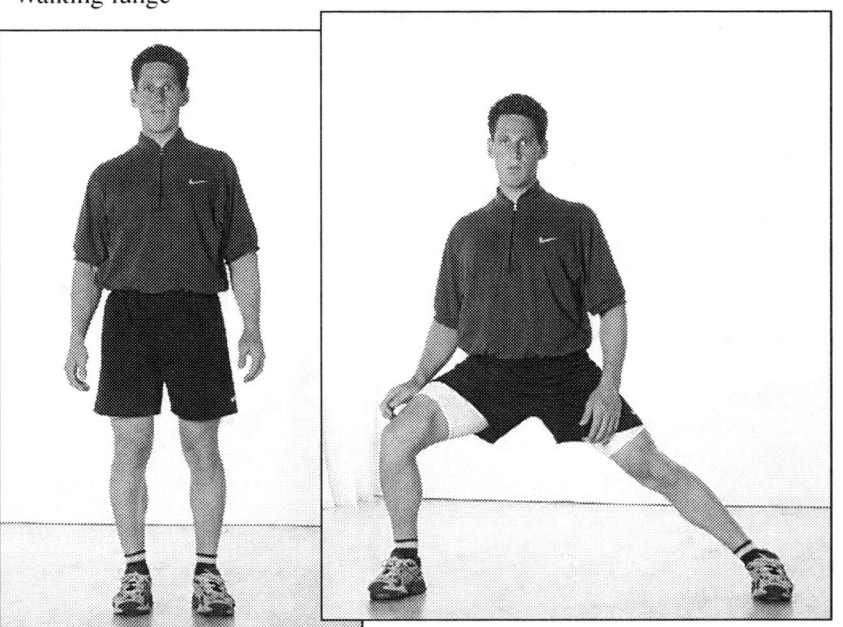

Figure 3.75
Side lunge

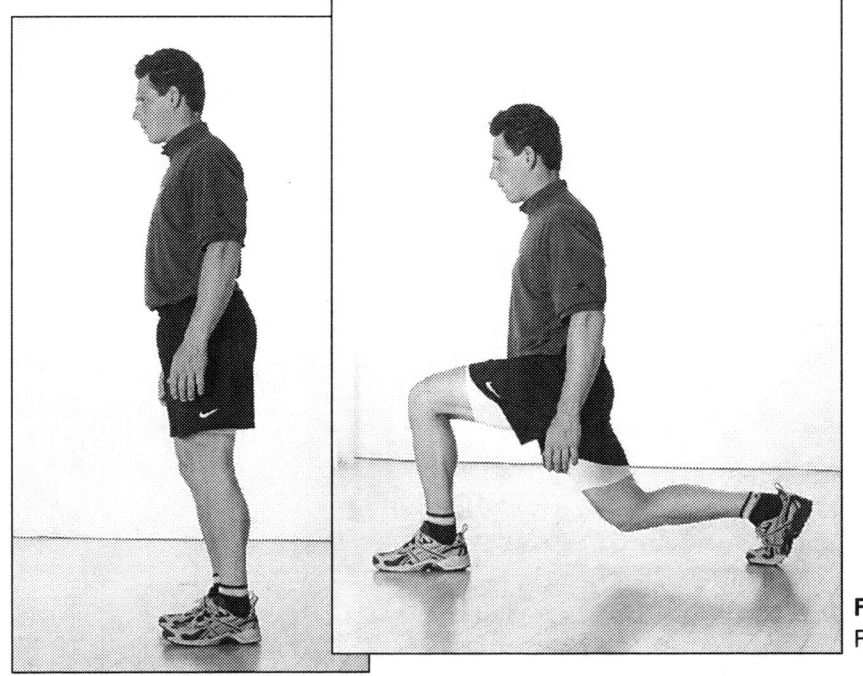

Figure 3.76
Front lunge

Hip Extension

Targeted muscle: Glutes, hamstrings

Starting position: Lie in a prone position with arms folded and head resting on the arms so that a neutral spine can be maintained (Figure 3.77).

Action: Leading with the heel, slowly raise one leg up toward the ceiling (Figure 3.78). Pause, then slowly return to the starting position. Repeat with the other leg.

Common errors:

Error: Lifting the head

Correction: Keep the head and neck aligned with the spine.

Error: Arching the lower back

Correction: Do not raise the exercising leg too high.

Variation:

• Prone on bench

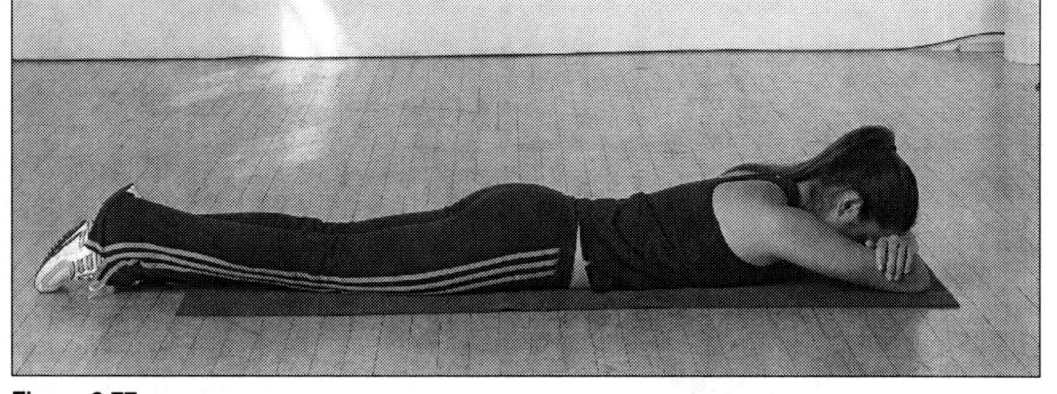

Figure 3.77
Hip extension; starting position

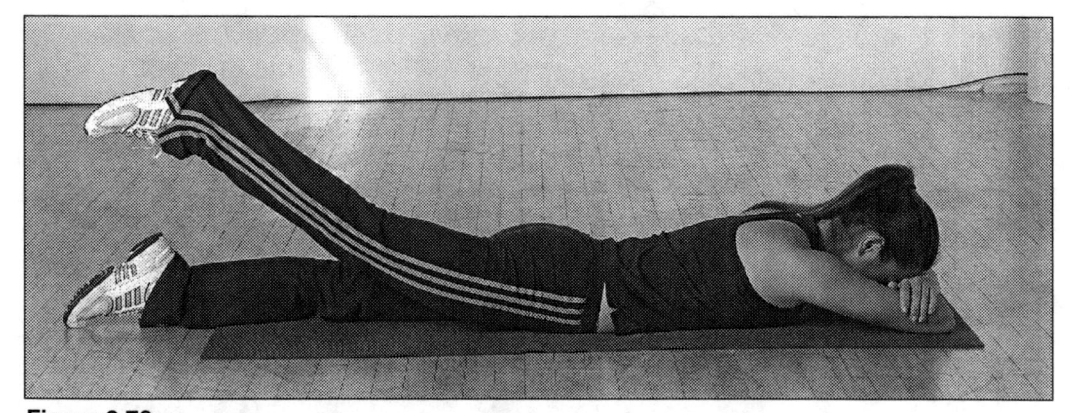

Figure 3.78
Hip extension; action

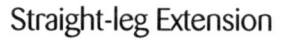
Straight-leg Extension

Targeted muscle: Iliopsoas

Starting position: Sit on a bench with one leg bent and the other extended. Engage the abdominals to help stabilize the spine and pelvis (Figure 3.79).

Action: Keep the leg extended and slowly raise the straight leg (Figure 3.80). Pause, then slowly return to the starting position. Repeat with the other leg.

Variations:

• Standing

• To decrease intensity, shorten the length of the lever by bending the knee of the leg being lifted.

Equipment variation:

• Elastic resistance (seated or standing)

Common error:

Error: Leaning back with the trunk while lifting the leg

Correction: Maintain an upright neutral spine by engaging the abdominals and equally distributing the body weight on the buttocks.

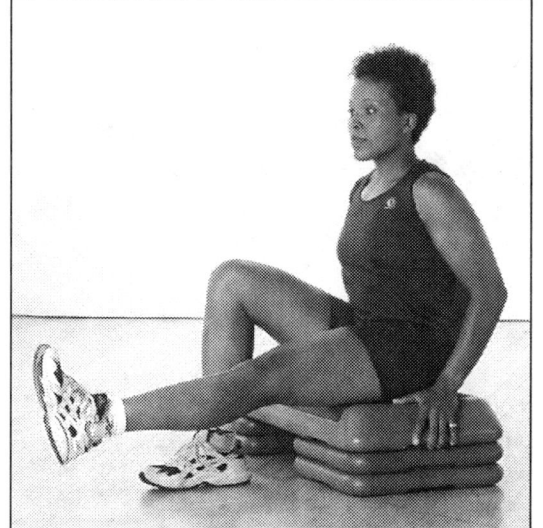

Figure 3.79
Straight-leg extension; starting position

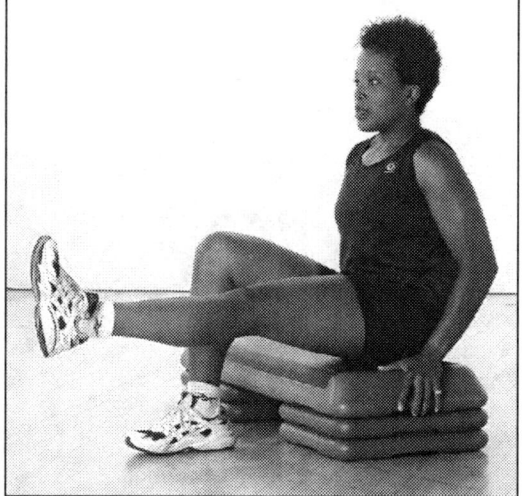

Figure 3.80
Straight-leg extension; action

Outer Thigh Lift

Targeted muscles: Hip abductors

Starting position: Lie on the left side and rest the head on the arm, keeping the neck in line with the rest of the spine. Bend the left leg and engage the abdominals to help stabilize the spine and pelvis. Keep the right leg extended and toes pointed forward (Figure 3.81).

Action: Abduct the leg through a full range of motion (Figure 3.82). Pause, then slowly return to the starting position. Repeat with the other leg.

Variations:

• Standing

• To decrease intensity, shorten the length of the lever by bending the knee of the leg being lifted.

Equipment variation:

• Elastic resistance (standing or side-lying)

Common errors:

Error: Allowing the hips to roll forward or backward while performing the exercise

Correction: Maintain a neutral pelvis by engaging the abdominals and stabilizing the pelvis, not allowing it to move during execution of the exercise.

Error: Allowing the thigh to externally rotate while lifting the leg

Correction: Keep the knee facing forward throughout the exercise.

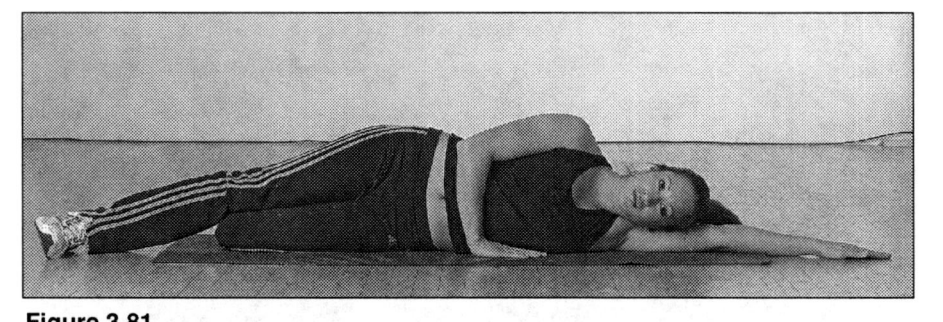

Figure 3.81
Outer thigh lift; starting position

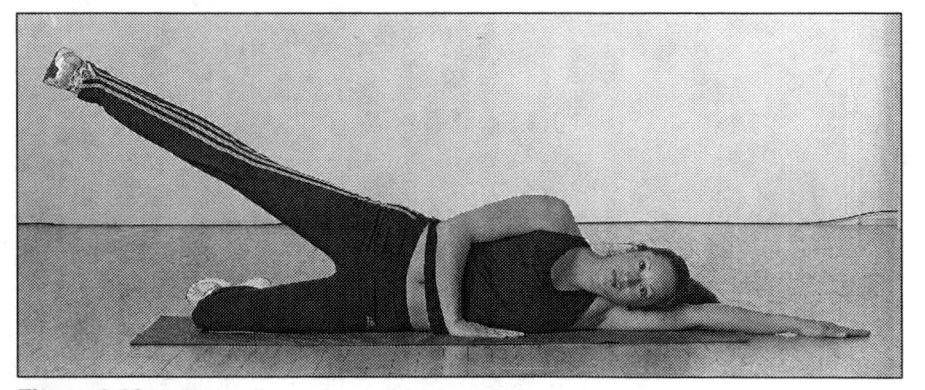

Figure 3.82
Outer thigh lift; action

Inner Thigh Lift

Targeted muscles: Hip adductors

Starting position: Lie on the left side, and rest the head on the arm, keeping the neck in line with the rest of the spine. Hips and shoulders should face forward with the abdominals engaged to help stabilize the spine and pelvis. Straighten the lower leg, then bend and cross the upper leg over it (Figure 3.83).

Action: Slowly lift the lower leg through a full range of motion (Figure 3.84). Pause, then slowly return to the starting position. Repeat with the other leg.

Variations:

• To decrease intensity, shorten the length of the lever by bending the knee of the leg being lifted.

• Supine; flex both hips 90 degrees. From an adducted position, slowly abduct the thighs and return to the starting position.

Equipment variation:

• Elastic resistance (standing or side-lying)

Common errors:

Error: Allowing the hips to roll forward or backward while performing the exercise

Correction: Maintain a neutral pelvis by engaging the abdominals and stabilizing the pelvis, and not allowing it to move during execution of the exercise.

Error: Allowing the thigh to externally rotate while lifting the leg

Correction: Keep the lower knee facing forward throughout the exercise.

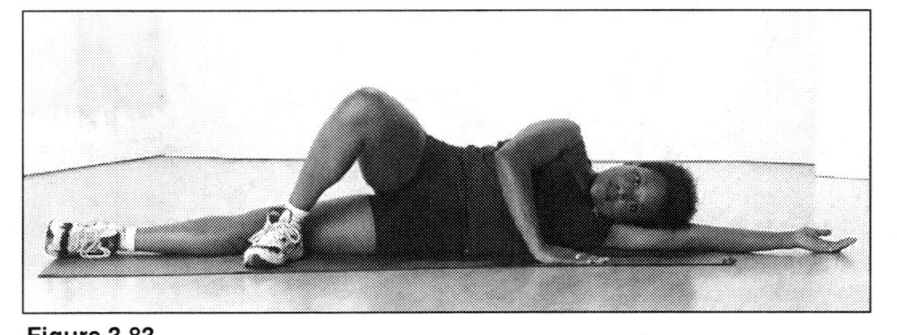

Figure 3.83
Inner thigh lift; starting position

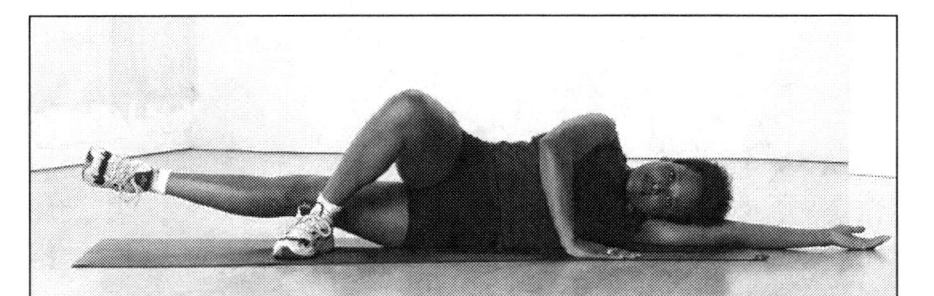

Figure 3.84
Inner thigh lift; action

Lower Legs

Muscles involved: Gastrocnemius, soleus, anterior tibialis

Strength-training technique for the lower leg: During heel raises, especially on a step or bench, use a wall or weighted bar for added stability.

Heel Raise

Targeted muscles: Gastrocnemius, soleus

Starting position: Start with feet shoulder-width apart, knees slightly bent, and engage the abdominals to help support the lower back (Figure 3.85).

Action: Plantarflex up on the toes (Figure 3.86). Pause, then slowly lower to the starting position.

Table 3.8
Exercises for the Lower Legs

Position	Resistance	Exercises
Standing	Weights	Heel raise
Standing	Bodyweight	Heel raise
Seated	Bodyweight	Toe raise

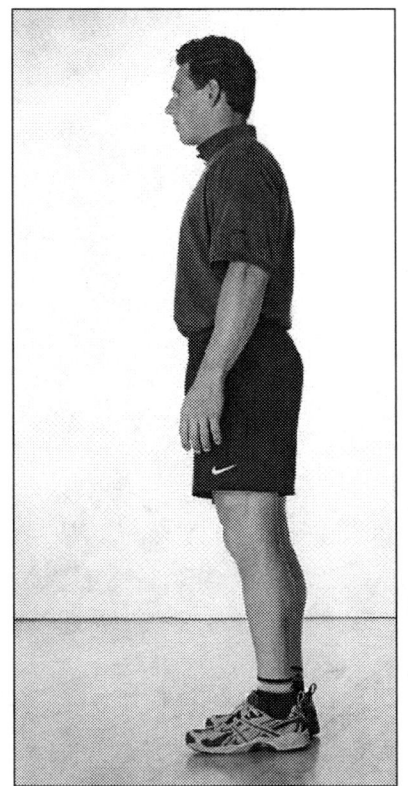

Figure 3.85
Heel raise; starting position

Figure 3.86
Heel raise; action

Variation:

• One foot at a time, hanging the heel of the working leg off the edge of a bench while the other leg maintains full contact with the bench (Figure 3.87).

Equipment variations:

• Dumbbells held at waist or shoulder level

• Weighted bar held on top of the shoulders

Common error:

Error: Leaning forward with the trunk while lifting the heels

Correction: Maintain a neutral spine by engaging the abdominals and stabilizing the spine, and not allowing the hips to move during execution of the exercise.

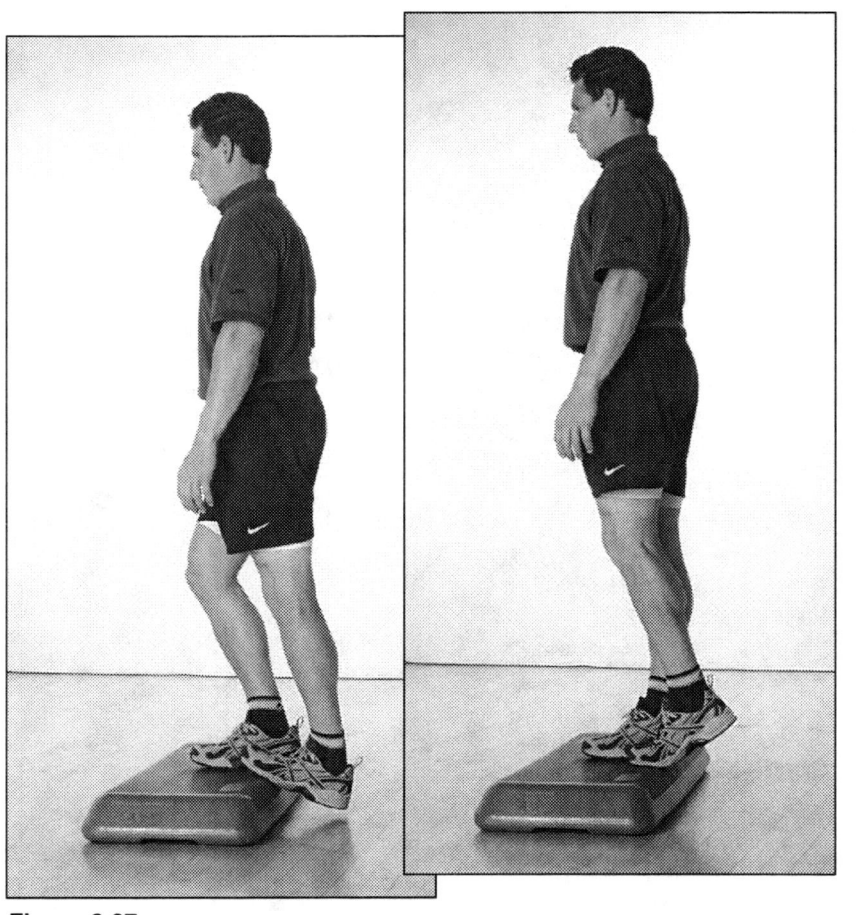

Figure 3.87
Heel raises variation; using a step

Toe Raise

Targeted muscle: Anterior tibialis

Starting position: In a seated position, place one foot on top of the other (Figure 3.88).

Action: Dorsiflex against the resistance applied by the non-working foot (Figure 3.89).

Variation:

• Rotate the foot inward and outward to work different aspects of the anterior shin.

Equipment variation:

• Strap a light ankle weight around the middle of the foot.

Common error:

Error: Leaning back with the trunk while lifting the foot

Correction: Maintain an upright neutral spine by engaging the abdominals and equally distributing the body weight on the buttocks.

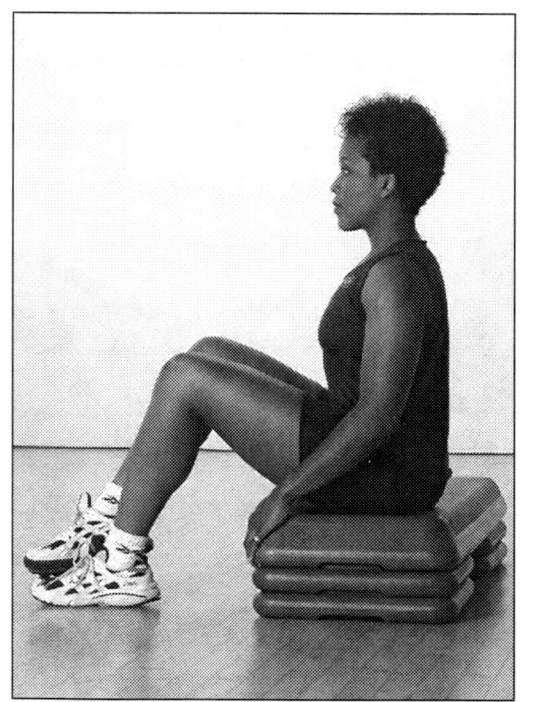

Figure 3.88
Toe raise; starting position

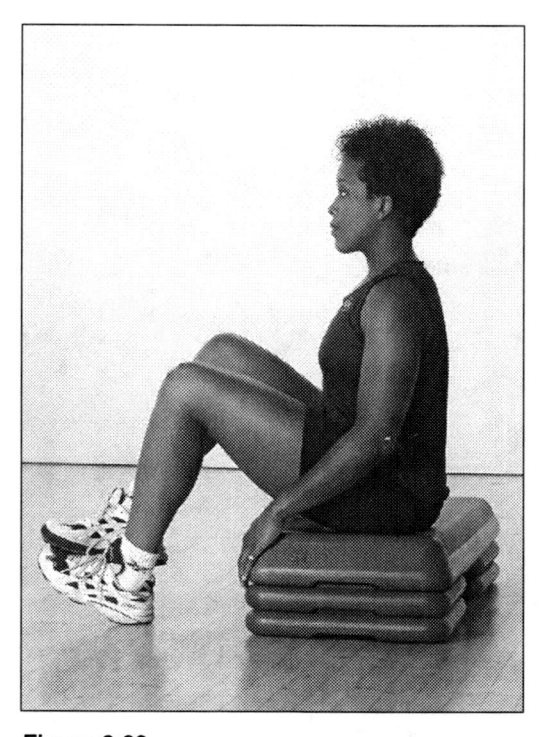

Figure 3.89
Toe raise; action

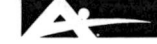
Teaching a Group Strength Training Class

CHAPTER FOUR

Verbal Introduction

Before beginning class, introduce yourself, the class or class format, and review some safety reminders relevant to the class. Encourage participants to tell you if they are feeling discomfort with any specific exercise or movement pattern. This should also prepare participants for the one-on-one feedback given during class.

"Good morning. My name is Chris. Welcome to the Upper-body Design Class. Before we get started I wanted to remind you to go at your own pace throughout the class. We can always adjust the resistance, the exercise, or your alignment to make the exercises work for you. I will be circulating through the class so that I can provide you with feedback to keep you exercising effectively.

Please do the following:

If you feel any sharp or sudden pain, stop and let me know.

Drink plenty of water.

Take breaks when necessary."

Risk Assessment

On any given day, a new participant can enter a group fitness class and be a walking time bomb. The participant may have advanced coronary disease, **arthritis,** or severe low-back pain. When placed in a group situation, the participant may not disclose his or her medical history to you. Moreover, a regular participant may develop a condition that poses new challenges to completing a strength-training class.

For these reasons, it is vitally important to screen participants during the introduction before class starts. Some participants may even require a medical screening prior to exercising.

Speak to new participants individually. Exchange simple information, such as names and commonalities. Ask the individual if he or she has any medical concerns, medications, or musculoskeletal challenges that need to be discussed. Also, ask if participants have any changes in their health status that need to be addressed. If a participant has not already completed informed consent and health history forms, have them do so for your records.

Guidelines for New Students

It is your job to make new students feel as if they are part of the group. Follow these tips to attract and keep new participants.

1. *Welcome new students.* Greet them with a smile and thank them for attending your class.

2. *Review medical history.* You will want to know if there are any special precautions you need to offer during class.

3. *Set class expectations.* Review some of the main points of the class (e.g., the class format, main goals of the class).

4. *Create a sense of community.* Introduce each new student to other participants so that everyone can learn his or her name.

5. *Check their progress.* Let participants know that you will be coming over to them throughout the class to make sure they are comfortable.

6. *Acknowledge the participants.* Make eye contact, smile, and offer kudos for a job well done.

7. *Provide feedback sensitively.* You may want to walk over to new participants and offer feedback on form without drawing too much attention.

8. *Include new students in discussions and stories.* To help new students feel like they are part of the group, avoid telling jokes or stories that only the regular students know about.

9. *Improve program adherence.* Encourage new students to come back for your next class.

10. *Ask new students for feedback.* Let them know that they have input on how the class is taught. For example, "Are there any other exercises you would like to see during the class?"

Technique Review

Proper exercise execution can only occur if participants are in the proper starting position. A simple method for guiding participants into proper alignment is using either a toe-to-head or head-to-toe approach. Using this method, you can ensure that the key areas of the body are guided into proper alignment. As cues are given, begin at one end of the body and work toward the other end of the body. Following are examples of guiding participants into abdominal curls using the two different methods. Note that the cues are the same, but the order is different.

Head-to-toe: Support your head with the palms of your hands, elbows to the side, neutral spine, one knee bent and the other leg extended.

Toe-to-head: One knee bent and the other leg extended, neutral spine, support your head with the palms of your hands, and elbows to the side.

Cueing

Cueing helps participants understand how the exercise should be performed as well as what to do next. There are three different categories of cues offered during class.

1. Movement cues initiate movements and/or modify existing movements.
   For example: "three up and one down; single arm only; front, then side"

2. Motivational cues help increase the motivation and effort of the participants.
   For example: "squeeze," "getting stronger," or "almost done"

3. Safety and alignment cues help improve the performance of the exercise.
   For example: "keep your knee over your ankle" or "support your lower back by placing one hand on your mid-thigh"

Types of Feedback

There are four components to a complete feedback statement. Use them individually or in sequence.

Knowledge of Results

This type of feedback is a nonjudgmental statement that simply informs the participant of what you are observing. Some examples of knowledge of results feedback are:

"Your knee has gone past your toes."

"Your lower back is arched excessively."

The purpose of this type of feedback is to act like a mirror. Describe the performance, good or bad, of the participant. Ultimately, participants must learn to recognize when they are performing the movement incorrectly.

Corrective

This type of feedback states the correct method of performance. It lets participants know the specific performance that is required. Some examples of corrective feedback are:

"Exhale during the exertion."

"Move your knee above your ankle."

"Keep the spine neutral."

This type of feedback may also include statements that can help participants learn to regulate their own performance. For example, explain that when the knee moves forward past the ankle it blocks the view of the shoelaces. In this way, the participant can begin to self-regulate performance.

Confirming

This type of feedback lets participants know when they have performed the movement correctly. Some examples of this type of feedback are:

"That's the way!"

"You got it!"

"That's right!"

Instructional

This type of feedback offers the explanation or rationale behind the feedback. Participants can fully understand the importance and consequences of their performances. With greater understanding of the rationale, compliance and motivation will increase. For example, explain that holding the breath during strength-training exercises can elevate blood pressure. Therefore, an established breathing pattern can reduce an elevation in blood pressure.

Intensity Monitoring

Make every effort to walk around the entire room. Besides the benefit of giving each person an acknowledgment, this gives you an opportunity to monitor intensity and performance.

As mentioned above, it has been shown that when a participant holds his or her breath during strenuous exercise there is an increased elevation in blood pressure. Although most instructors urge participants to exhale during the lifting phase of an exercise, a relaxed breathing pattern during the lowering phase is equally effective.

Monitor each participant to ensure that he or she is not holding the breath. A red or strenuous look

---

Feedback Statements

There are three types of strategies for giving feedback statements during class.

1. The overhead statement is not directed at any one person and is offered to the entire class. This is useful when you see incorrect form in more than one participant and do not want to draw attention to any single individual.
2. The proximal statement is made for the benefit of all participants, but with one or two individuals in mind. Move close to the participant or participants that require feedback. Do not directly face the participant, but place yourself in the participant's personal space; it is most effective when you are in the direct line of view of the participant.
3. The direct statement is made directly to the participant who requires feedback. Although some participants may feel awkward with this approach, it is necessary to ensure the exercises are performed safely and effectively.

on a participant's face may be an indication that the individual needs to breathe more regularly.

To Touch or Not to Touch

One-on-one training can occur in a group setting. As you move around the room monitoring participants, one-on-one instruction inevitably takes place. Use discretion and always ask permission prior to touching any participants. A simple question, May I touch your shoulder to help teach you the movement? will let you know how comfortable the participant is with touching.

The value of using touch is tremendous and is a highly effective teaching tool. There are two strategies you can use: the "hands-on" method and the "hands-off" method.

Example: You are leading a single-arm triceps kick-back using weights and notice that a participant's elbow is dropping during the movement rather than remaining stationary.

Hands-on: Place your palm or the back of your hand in the correct spot for the elbow. Instruct the participant to keep contact with the hand for the entire range of motion. When the elbow drifts off the hand, the participant feels the change and begins to become more aware of the error (Figure 4.1).

Hands-off: Place the participant's elbow in the correct starting position, then place your own hand about one inch below the participant's upper arm near the elbow, but without touching it. When the participant's elbow drops, they feel your hand, which helps them become more aware of the error (Figure 4.2).

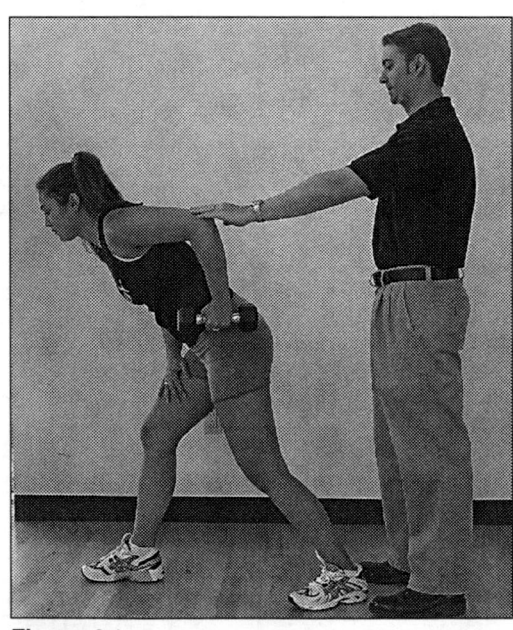

Figure 4.1
The "hands-on" method; single-arm triceps kick-back

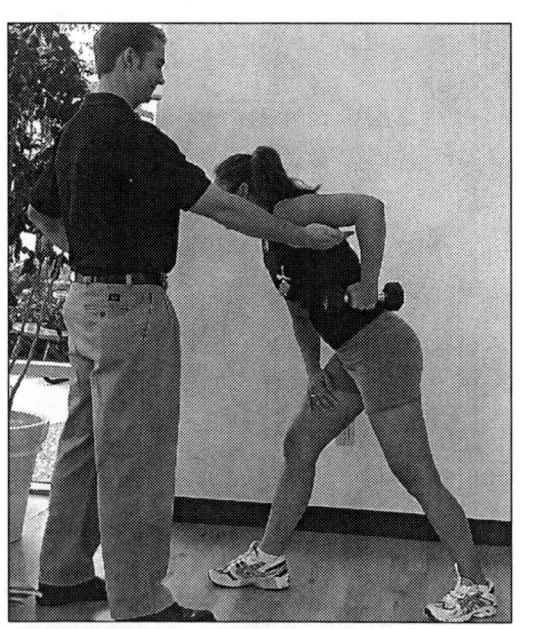

Figure 4.2
The "hands-off" method; single-arm triceps kick-back

Injury Prevention

To avoid injury to the spine and back muscles, teach participants to maintain a neutral spinal alignment, which is the position in which the spine is best equipped to deal with external stress and strain. Unlike other exercises that are specific to the classroom, postural maintenance is performed throughout the day.

When teaching in a room with mirrors, have participants view their spinal alignment from the side so they can become more aware of their alignment.

It is estimated that close to 80% of the population will suffer an episode of lower-back pain at some point in their lives. Therefore, avoid placing excessive stress on the lower back and be aware if any of your participants have a history of lower-back pain.

Establishing Range-of-Motion Limits

Some exercises have established range-of-motion (ROM) limits, or stopping points. Movement that goes beyond this point can cause injury. Identify these ROM limits prior to starting the exercise. In this way, participants can increase their awareness of the crucial position.

For example, during the supine chest fly exercise, it is common for participants to lower the arms too fast, which causes the arms to drop too low. Remedy this by establishing the lower range of motion as the starting point. Lifting up from the starting point and then emphasizing the slow and controlled lowering of the arms can help avoid moving beyond the safe limits of the exercise.

Table 4.1
Postural Deviations and Associated Muscle Imbalances

Malalignment	Possible Tight Muscles	Possible Weak Muscles
Excessive lordosis	Lower back (erectors), hip flexors	Internal obliques, rectus abdominis, hip extensors
Flat-back	Rectus abdominis, hip extensors	Lower back (erectors), hip flexors
Sway-back	Rectus abdominis, hip flexors	Obliques, lower rectus abdominis, hip extensors
Excessive kyphosis	Rectus abdominis, internal obliques, shoulder adductors, internal rotators (pectorals and latissimus), intercostals	Erector spinae of the thoracic spine, scapular adductors (mid and lower trapezius)
Forward neck	Cervical flexors, upper trapezius	Neck extensors

Modifications

There are three ways to modify strength-training intensity: external resistance, lever changes (modifying the body position to work against gravity), and active rest.

External Resistance

To increase the intensity, increase the resistance (e.g., increase the weight, shorten the band, choose a band with greater resistance, or add manual resistance). To decrease the intensity, reduce the resistance (e.g., reduce the weight, lengthen the band, or choose a band with less resistance).

Lever Changes

To decrease intensity, shorten the lever by bending the elbows or placing the weight closer to the joint that is moving. To increase intensity, lengthen the lever or move the weight farther from the joint that is moving.

Active Rest

To increase the intensity, decrease the amount of rest between sets or between repetitions. To decrease intensity, perform fewer repetitions by alternating between right and left sides or by alternating between lifting and resting.

For example, lateral deltoid raises can be modified to reduce the intensity in the following ways:

1. Reduce the weight being lifted.
2. Bend the elbow 90 degrees.
3. Alternate between right and left sides or between lateral raises and biceps curls.

In addition to intensity modifications, you may need to offer modifications to reduce the stress on the lower back.

Overhead exercises can be performed with one arm at a time to reduce the stress on the spine. Bent-over and upright exercises can be modified into a staggered stance with one leg forward and one leg backward. The hand that is on the same side as the forward leg is placed on the upper thigh for support. This leaves the other hand free for single-arm exercises.

On the floor, extended legs can decrease the mobility of the pelvis and encourage poor posture. Bend one knee and bring the foot closer to the hips to support the back.

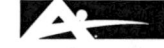

Programming

CHAPTER FIVE

Warm-up

Each strength-training class should begin with a gradual warm-up to psychologically and physically prepare participants for the workout. The focus of the warm-up should be on joint preparation and rehearsal of movements to be used in class.

Cool-down

Because blood tends to accumulate in the lower body when vigorous exercise is stopped abruptly, lower-intensity exercises are recommended to facilitate active recovery. As a general guideline, the last five to 10 minutes of the class should be dedicated to cool-down activity.

Always make sure that participants have fully recovered and are below 60% of maximum heart rate before transitioning to a floor position. Quickly moving from a standing to lying position causes pooled blood to rush toward the heart. Participants with compromised cardiovascular systems should be particularly cautious as this can lead to heart attacks or other failures of the cardio-vascular system.

Exercise Sequencing

There are three formats used to sequence exercises into a class: (1) upper/lower, (2) large to small, and (3) agonist/antagonist.

Plan transitions so starting positions (standing vs. floor) and equipment variations (weights vs. elastic resistance) are closely related. Avoid changing both starting position and equipment at one time.

Upper/Lower

In this format, alternate between upper- and lower-body exercises, allowing ample recovery time for each body part.

Sample class

Standing

Elastic

Chest press

Outer thigh lift

Single-arm lat pull-down

Inner thigh lift

Weights

Lateral deltoid raise

Heel raise

Triceps kick-back

Squat

Biceps curl

Bodyweight

Front lunge

Prone

Bodyweight

Push-up

Hip extension

Seated

Bodyweight

Bench dip

Toe raise

Weights

Biceps curl

Bodyweight

Straight leg extension

Elastic

Internal shoulder extension

Abdominal/torso exercises

Abdominal curl

Side bridge

Single-leg reverse curl

Back extension

End class with a cool-down stretch routine.

Each pair of exercises can be a performed as a single set or in a two-set format.

Large to Small

This format begins with large muscle groups of the legs and works progressively toward the

smaller muscle groups of the torso and arms. Participants work the larger muscle groups when they are least fatigued.

Plan transitions so starting positions (standing vs. floor) and equipment variations (weights vs. elastic resistance) are closely related. Avoid changing both starting position and equipment at one time.

Sample Class

Quads, Hamstrings, & Gluteals

Squats (Standing/Bodyweight)

Walking lunges (Standing/Bodyweight)

Abductors

Outer thigh lift (Side-lying/Bodyweight)

Adductors

Inner thigh lift (Side-lying/Bodyweight)

Torso

Side bridge (Side-lying/Bodyweight)

Abdominal curl (Supine/Bodyweight)

Back extensors

Back extension (Prone/Bodyweight)

Chest

Push-up (Prone/Bodyweight)

Back

Scapular retraction (All-fours/Weights)

Shoulders

Overhead press (Standing/Weights)

Lateral deltoid raise (Standing/Weights)

Biceps

Biceps curl (Standing/Weights)

Triceps

Triceps kick-back (Standing/Weights)

End class with a cool-down stretch routine.

Each pair of exercises can be a performed as a single set or in a two-set format.

Agonist/Antagonist

This format works opposing muscle groups in pairs. This helps prevent muscle imbalances caused by strengthening only one muscle group.

Sample Class

Chest/Back

Weights: Chest fly / Single-arm bent row

Elastic resistance: Chest press / Seated row

Shoulders

Weights: Front deltoid raise / Posterior shoulder extension

Elastic resistance: Single-arm Arnold press / Posterior shoulder extension

Biceps/Triceps

Weights: Biceps curl / Overhead triceps press

Elastic resistance: Seated biceps curl / Triceps kick-back

Torso

Bodyweight: Abdominal curl / Back extension

Quadriceps/Hamstrings

Bodyweight: Backward lunge / Hip extension

Hip abductors / Hip adductors

Elastic resistance: Outer thigh lift / Inner thigh lift

Plantarflexors / Dorsiflexors

Bodyweight: Heel raises / Toe raises

Each pair of exercises can be a performed as a single set or in a two-set format.

Group Circuit Class

A circuit class provides cardiovascular-endurance training along with muscular-endurance training. The circuit can be modified to meet the fitness level of the participants as well as space, equipment, and time limitations.

Sample Class: Combo Circuit Class

Fitness level: Moderate to advanced

Time: 45 minutes (set-up and break-down time is not included)

Music tempo: 120–130 bpm

Class size: Provide one piece of equipment per station for each group of 15 participants. A class size of 16 to 30 participants requires two pieces of equipment at each station.

Equipment: Station equipment, stop watch, whistle, and towel (to clean sweat on equipment or on floor)

Directions: Set up 15 stations around the room (Figure 5.1). Place a sign at each station that indicates the name and number of the exercise within the sequence. For example, the sign for the first station would display "#1-Push-up."

After a five-minute warm-up, instruct each participant to move to a station. Provide beginners with a buddy who can help them work through the circuit and place them at station #1 to make the circuit easier to understand.

For the first minute, each participant performs a station exercise. Using the stop watch, indicate the 30-second mark and the 50-second mark (10 seconds left.) You can also prepare a tape recording that alternates between 60 seconds of music and 20 to 30 seconds of silence to indicate transition time between stations.

Blow the whistle to signal the movement of the class to the next station in the circuit. After 15 minutes, each station has been performed once. After 30 minutes, or two complete cycles, begin the cool-down. A five-minute cool-down followed by five minutes of stretching allows for proper recovery.

Variations: Use cardio equipment, bikes, rowing machines, or trampolines. Add sports-specific exercises (e.g., power leaps and hops). Add a 15- to 30-second transition exercise, such as jumping jacks or shuffle exercises, in between the stations.

Music

Select music to make the class fun and enjoyable for all participants. To ensure the exercises are performed slowly and with control, the music's **beats** per minute (bpm) should fall within the range of 110–130 bpm. When the tempo of the music is faster than 130 bpm, there is a tendency for alignment and form to decline. This is especially true for beginning participants. Music that is extremely fast, above 180 bpm,

Figure 5.1

Group Circuit Class

Station #	Exercise	Equipment
1	push-ups	exercise mat
2	sit-ups	exercise mat
3	pull-ups	pull-up bar in doorway / exercise band
4	side bridges	exercise mat
5	front deltoid raises	dumbbell or bands
6	bouncing	mini-trampoline
7	side deltoid raises	dumbbell or exercise band
8	jump rope	jump rope
9	biceps curls	dumbbell or exercise band
10	jumping jacks	
11	triceps curls	dumbbell or exercise band
12	step (over the top*)	step or bench
13	squats	dumbbell or exercise band
14	towel jumps	towel or a line of masking tape on floor
15	walking lunges	dumbbell

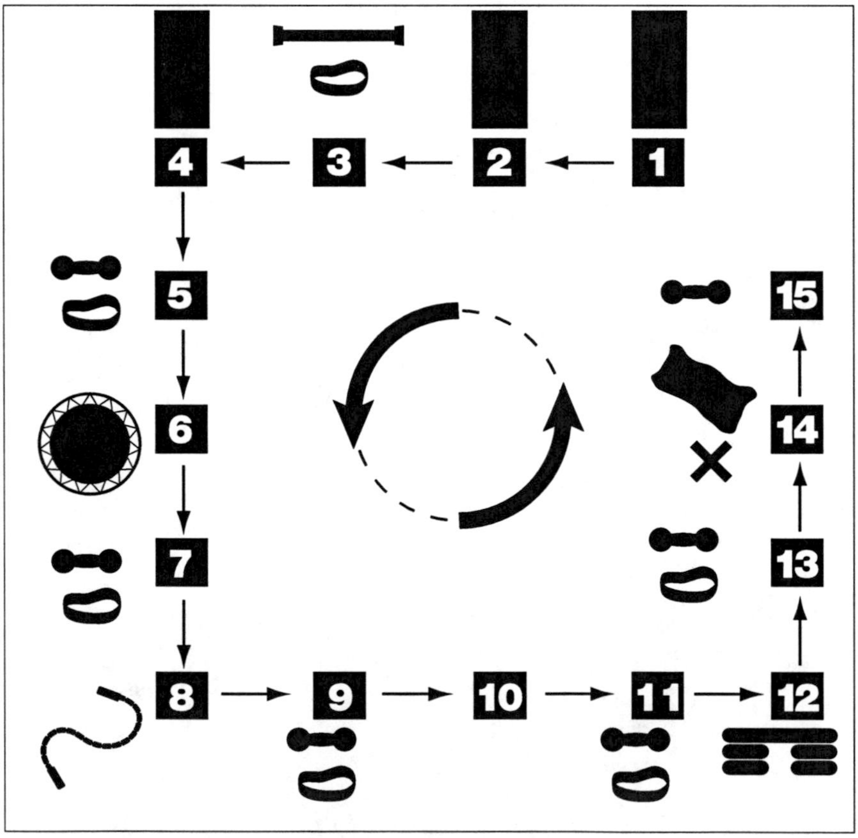

*When performing step training, choose alternating exercises to work both sides of the body, or exercise 30 seconds on one leg and 30 seconds on the other.

can be performed at half time (i.e., moving to every other beat of the music) to compensate.

Because music influences the way people perform the exercises, it is also recommended that the concentric muscle action is placed with the downbeat, or on the "1 count." For example, when abdominal curls are done so the eccentric muscle action is placed with the downbeat, participants tend to accelerate through the eccentric phase rather than controlling the movement.

Agonist – A muscle that is directly engaged in contraction; opposes the action of an antagonist muscle.

Antagonist – A muscle that acts in opposition to the action produced by an agonist.

Applied Force – An external force acting on a system (body or body segment).

Arthritis – Inflammatory condition involving a joint.

Beats – Regular pulsations that have an even rhythm and occur in a continuous pattern of strong and weak pulsations.

Body Composition – The makeup of the body in terms of percentage of lean body mass and body fat.

Bursitis – Irritation of a bursa, which is a padlike fluid-filled sac located at friction sites throughout the body; bursitis occurs most often in the knees, hips, shoulders, and elbows.

Calisthenics – Exercises to increase muscular strength or endurance that use the weight of the body or body parts for resistance.

Chondromalacia – A gradual softening and degeneration of the articular cartilage, usually involving the back surface of the patella (knee cap). This condition may produce pain and swelling, or a grinding sound or sensation when the knee is flexed and extended.

Concentric – A muscle action in which the muscle shortens.

Contraindication – Any condition that renders some particular movement, activity, or treatment improper or undesirable.

Cueing – A visual or verbal technique, using hand signals or a few words, to inform exercise participants of upcoming movements.

Eccentric – A muscle action in which the muscle lengthens against a resistance while producing force.

Extension – Movement that increases the angle between two bones of a joint, such as straightening of the elbow.

Flexion – The movement that decreases the angle between two bones of a joint.

Force Arm – The lever arm length (the perpendicular distance from the axis to the line of the force) of the motive force.

Isometric – Muscular contraction in which there is no change in the angle of the involved joint(s) and little or no change in the length of the contracting muscle.

Kinesiology – The study of the principles of mechanics and anatomy in relation to human movement.

Lever – A rigid bar that rotates around a fixed support (fulcrum) in response to an applied force.

Low-back Pain (LBP) – A general term to describe a multitude of back conditions, including muscular and ligament strains, sprains, and injuries. The cause of LBP is often elusive; most LBP is probably caused by muscle imbalance and weakness.

Motive Force –The force that starts or causes a movement.

Muscular Endurance – The ability of a muscle or muscle group to exert force against a resistance over a sustained period of time.

Muscular Strength – The maximal force a muscle or muscle group can exert during a single contraction.

Strength Training – The process of exercising with progressively heavier resistance for the purpose of strengthening the musculoskeletal system.

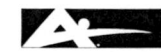

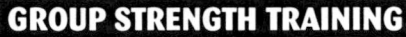

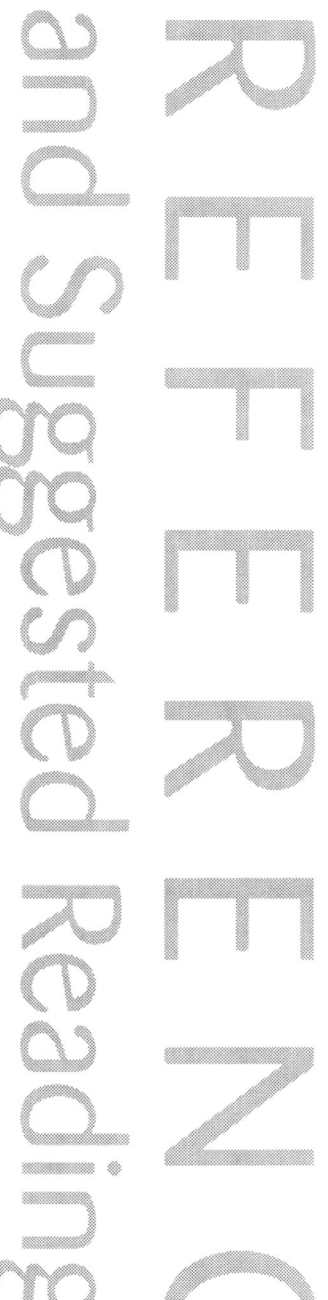

Alter, M.J. (1996). *Science of Flexibility* (2nd ed.). Champaign, Ill.: Human Kinetics.

American Council on Exercise (2003). *ACE Personal Trainer Manual* (3rd ed.). San Diego: American Council on Exercise.

American Council on Exercise (2000). *Group Fitness Instructor Manual.* San Diego: American Council on Exercise.

Baechle, T.R. & Earle, R.W. (2000). *Essentials of Strength Training and Conditioning* (2nd ed.). Champaign, Ill.: Human Kinetics.

Brooks, D. (1993). *Theory and Mechanics of Resistance Training.* Mammoth Lakes, Calif.: Moves International.

Clarke, D.H. (1975). *Exercise Physiology.* Englewood Cliffs, N.J.: Prentice Hall Inc.

Crisco, J. & Panjabi, M.M. (1991). The intersegmental and multiseg-mental muscles of the lumbar spine. *Spine,* 16, 793–799.

Ellison, D. (1995). Exercise for function, part one. *IDEA Today,* March, 13, 3.

Ellison, D. (1995). Exercise for function, part two. *IDEA Today,* April, 13, 4.

Hall, T., David, A., Geere, J., & Salvenson, K. (1995). *Relative recruitment of the abdominal muscles during three levels of exertion during abdominal hollowing.* Gold Coast, Queensland: Manipulative Physiotherapists Association of Australia.

Hedrick, A. (1995). Training for hypertrophy. *Strength and Conditioning,* 17, 2, 22–29.

Hodges, P.W. & Richardson, C.A. (1995). Neuromotor dysfunction of the trunk musculature in low back pain patients. In: *Proceedings of the International Congress of the World Confederation of Physical Therapists.* Washington, D.C.

Hodges, P.W. & Richardson, C.A. (1996). Inefficient muscular stabilization of the lumbar spine associated with low back pain. *Spine,* 21, 22, 2640–2650.

Hodges, P.W., Richardson, C.A., & Jull, G. (1996). Evaluation of the relationship between laboratory and clinical tests of transverse abdominis function. *Physiotherapy Research International,* 1, 30–40.

Lacourse, M.G. (1994). Touching for strength. *IDEA Today,* May, 12, 5.

Richardson, C.A, Jull, G., Hodges, P.W., & Hides, J.A. (1999). *Therapeutic Exercise for Spinal Segmental Stabilization in Low Back Pain.* New York: Churchill Livingstone.

Wescott, W. (1994). *Strength Fitness* (4th ed.). Dubuque, Iowa: WCB/McGraw-Hill.

Wlodkowski, R.J. (1993). *Enhancing Adult Motivation to Learn.* San Francisco: Jossey Bass Publishers.

ABOUT THE AUTHOR

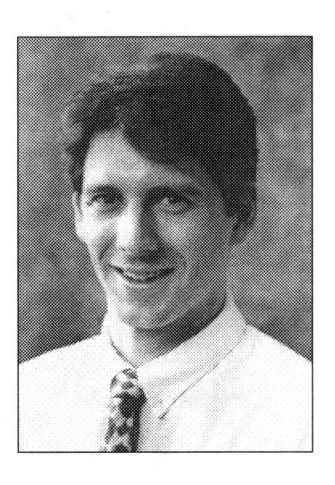

Richard J. Seibert, M.A., M.Ed., designs and delivers
training on leadership and service delivery for the
Department of the Navy. Seibert received his master's
degree in exercise physiology from the University of
Maryland, and later received a second master's degree in
education from the University of Massachusetts at Boston
in instructional design. He has combined these two disci-
plines to write study guides and articles, and create training
programs for fitness professionals. Seibert has been
teaching group fitness classes since 1987 and has presented
at fitness conventions around the world. As special projects
manager for ACE, he designed and delivered portions of
ACE's Group Exercise Practical Training Program.

Second edition
Copyright © 2004 American Council on Exercise (ACE)
Printed in the United States of America.

ABCDE

ISBN: 1-58518-903-0

Distributed by:
American Council on Exercise
P.O. Box 910449
San Diego, CA 92191-0449
(858) 279-8227
(858) 279-8064 (FAX)
www.ACEfitness.org

Managing Editor: Daniel J. Green
Technical Editor: Cedric X. Bryant, Ph.D.
Design & Production: Karen McGuire
Director of Publications: Christine J. Ekeroth
Assistant Editor: Jennifer Schiffer
Index: Bonny McLaughlin
Models: Paul Ainsworth, Valerie Gardner, and Giselle Pineda
Photography: Dennis Dal Covey

Acknowledgments:
Thanks to the entire American Council on Exercise staff for their support and guidance through the process of creating this manual.

NOTICE
The fitness industry is ever-changing. As new research and clinical experience broaden our knowledge, changes in programming and standards are required. The authors and the publisher of this work have checked with sources believed to be reliable in their efforts to provide information that is complete and generally in accord with the standards accepted at the time of publication. However, in view of the possibility of human error or changes in industry standards, neither the authors nor the publisher nor any other party who has been involved in the preparation or publication of this work warrants that the information contained herein is in every respect accurate or complete, and they are not responsible for any errors or omissions or the results obtained from the use of such information. Readers are encouraged to confirm the information contained herein with other sources.

Published by:
Healthy Learning Books & Videos
P.O. Box 1828
Monterey, CA 93942
(888) 229-5455
(831) 372-6075 (Fax)
www.healthylearning.com

P04-029

Group Strength Training

A Guide for Fitness Professionals from the American Council on Exercise

Second Edition

By Richard J. Seibert, M.A., M.Ed.

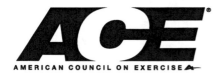

AMERICAN COUNCIL ON EXERCISE